Personal

DIET
JOURNAL

If found, please return to:

NAME ....

ADDRESS ....

PHONE NUMBER ....

EMAIL ADDRESS ....

STERLING
New York

An Imprint of Sterling Publishing
387 Park Avenue South
New York, NY 10016

ISBN 978-1-4549-1336-8

Distributed in Canada by Sterling Publishing
$c/_o$ Canadian Manda Group, 165 Dufferin Street
Toronto, Ontario, Canada M6K 3H6
Distributed in the United Kingdom by GMC Distribution Services
Castle Place, 166 High Street, Lewes, East Sussex, England BN7 1XU
Distributed in Australia by Capricorn Link (Australia) Pty. Ltd.
P.O. Box 704, Windsor, NSW 2756, Australia

For information about custom editions, special sales, and premium
and corporate purchases, please contact Sterling Special Sales
at 800-805-5489 or specialsales@sterlingpublishing.com.

Manufactured in China

4 6 8 10 9 7 5 3

www.sterlingpublishing.com

The groundwork
of all happiness
is health.

—LEIGH HUNT

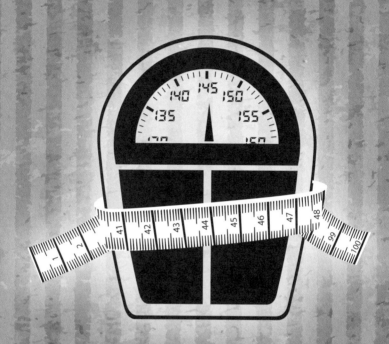

CONTENTS

Getting
HEALTHY

D id you know that about two-thirds of American adults are overweight? All those extra pounds not only make us feel self-conscious, but they can lead to serious health problems such as diabetes, high blood pressure, and even certain kinds of cancer. It's time to take your weight and measurements into your own hands and get healthy.

This journal is your all-inclusive guide to healthier living. It will help you set realistic and healthy goals for weight loss, track your diet and exercise progress, and keep you on the path to fitness and a healthier life

GOALS

The first step to weight loss is setting goals. On page 10 you will find a Body Mass Index, or BMI, chart that will show you a healthy weight for your height. Your goal weight should fall in the normal range. However, healthy weight loss averages 2 pounds per week, so don't set your goals too high, or too low. Your real goal is to discover a healthy lifestyle that will help you reach your desired weight and keep you there.

EATING

The next step is to understand your current eating behavior—and then to change it. To maintain your current weight you have to consume about 12 to 15 calories per day for every pound you weigh. So if you weigh 175 pounds, you need to eat 2,100 to 2,625 calories per day to stay there. If you want to lose weight, then you have to eat fewer calories. If you want to lose about 1 pound per week, you should reduce your calorie intake by about 500 calories per day. If you want to lose twice that, then you need to reduce your calorie intake by 1,000 calories per day. But don't push it too far! Women should eat at least 1,200 calories per day, and men should eat at least 1,500 to maintain a healthy diet.

Fats, carbohydrates, and protein are three of the most important energy producing nutrients for the human body, but that doesn't mean you should overdo it. Reducing the amount of fats and carbohydrates you eat is a great way to cut down on calorie consumption and promote healthy weight loss, because they are not only high in calories but low in vitamins and minerals, too.

To launch an overall healthier lifestyle, you should make sure you are getting all of the recommended vitamins and minerals and not eating "empty calories"—foods that have no nutritional value and are high in fat, carbs, and calories. Eating as little saturated fat as possible will lead to weight loss and healthy gains. Getting your daily protein from lean meats, cheese, yogurt, and eggs is a very healthy way to go, because each food has additional nutritional value above being high in protein.

To figure out your daily balance of calories and fats, use the formulas on pages 12–13.

At the back of this journal is a list of common foods, their calorie contents, and their fat contents. This guide will help you keep track of your daily fat and caloric intake when eating out or when you don't have a nutritional label on your food. Also included are charts that show the recommended intakes of vitamins and minerals, as well as lists of healthy foods that contain daily essentials. By using this information, you can construct a diet to help you lose weight, stay in good health, and eat foods you love.

WATER

People often overlook the importance of water in planning a healthy diet. There are numerous reasons why drinking water is great for everyone. People who drink eight 8-ounce glasses of water every day lose weight faster than people who don't, because water speeds up metabolic processes, helping you shed stored fat. It also moves waste and fat out of your body. Like oil in an engine, water keeps your body moving.

EXERCISE

The final step to a healthier you is exercise. Daily exercise will help you lose weight; strengthen your muscles, heart, and lungs; and give you more energy. Finding the right exercise for you is extremely important. First, take any health issues into consideration. Then, you need to find an aerobic activity that you enjoy. Exercise doesn't have to be a chore or a bore. Find a scenic place to walk, join a gym and learn karate, or discover that you're a natural tennis player. If you find an exercise you love, you'll stick with it and really enjoy your road to healthier living.

On pages 178–185 you will find a chart showing how many calories you burn per hour doing a variety of exercises.

A NEW YOU!

Leading a healthful life is the best thing you can do for yourself, and looking and feeling better for the rest of your life is within reach. Being conscious of the things you put into your body and do with your body is the only way to diet effectively and healthily. This journal will help you become aware of the things you're already doing that help or hurt you, and will guide you to better way of living. Get ready, because soon there will be a whole new you!

Body Mass Index

Your Body Mass Index (BMI)—calculated using your weight and height—is a fairly reliable assessment of proper weight and body fat. The formula for calculating your BMI is as follows:

FORMULA: WEIGHT (LB) / [HEIGHT (IN)]^2 X 703

BMI CATEGORIES:

Underweight = <18.5

Healthy weight = 18.5–24.9

Overweight = 25–29.9

Obese = BMI of 30 or greater

BMI Chart [1]

WEIGHT IN POUNDS

HEIGHT	HEALTHY WEIGHT						OVERWEIGHT					OBESE					
4'10"	91	96	100	105	110	115	119	124	129	134	138	143	148	153	158	162	167
4'11"	94	99	104	109	114	119	124	128	133	138	143	148	153	158	163	168	173
5'	97	102	107	112	118	123	128	133	138	143	148	153	158	163	158	174	179
5'1"	100	106	111	116	122	127	132	137	143	148	153	158	164	169	174	180	185
5'2"	104	109	115	120	126	131	136	142	147	153	158	164	169	175	180	186	191
5'3"	107	113	118	124	130	135	141	146	152	158	163	169	175	180	186	191	197
5'4"	110	116	122	128	134	140	145	151	157	163	169	174	180	186	192	197	204
5'5"	114	120	126	132	138	144	150	156	162	168	174	180	186	192	198	204	210
5'6"	118	124	130	136	142	148	155	161	167	173	179	186	192	198	204	210	216
5'7"	121	127	134	140	146	153	159	166	172	178	185	191	198	204	211	217	223
5'8"	125	131	138	144	151	158	164	171	177	184	190	197	203	210	216	223	230
5'9"	128	135	142	149	155	162	169	176	182	189	196	203	209	216	223	230	236
5'10"	132	139	146	153	160	167	174	181	188	195	202	209	216	222	229	236	243
5'11"	136	143	150	157	165	172	179	186	193	200	208	215	222	229	236	243	250
6'	140	147	154	162	169	177	184	191	199	206	213	221	228	235	242	250	258
6'1"	144	151	159	166	174	182	189	197	204	212	219	227	235	242	250	257	265
6'2"	148	155	163	171	179	186	194	202	210	218	225	233	241	249	256	264	272
6'3"	152	160	168	176	184	192	200	208	216	224	232	240	248	256	264	272	279
BMI	19	20	21	22	23	24	25	26	27	28	29	30	31	32	33	34	35

1. Body Mass Index Table
   U.S. Department of Health and Human Services
   National Institutes of Health
   nhlbi.nih.gov/guidelines/obesity/bmi_tbl.htm

GOALS

H ere is where your journal begins. List your goals—and not just the numbers! Write down how you expect to look and feel after the first month. Write down all the reasons you are starting a healthier lifestyle. Write down all the positive things you want to have happen as a result of a new and improved you!

WEIGHT

Healthy weight loss averages about two pounds per week. You may see more rapid results than this in the beginning, especially if you are more than 50 pounds overweight. To lose weight the right way and keep it off, pick a weight loss goal that is healthy and realistic.

10-WEEK GOAL:

Using the BMI chart, determine your Goal Weight.

GOAL WEIGHT:

CALORIES

To find the right **DAILY CALORIE BALANCE** for you, use the following formula:

Your weight x 15 (calories needed to maintain current weight) = current average calorie intake

Current average calorie intake – 500 = 1 lb. lost per week
Current average calorie intake – 750 = 1 – 1½ lb. lost per week
Current average calorie intake – 1000 = 2 lbs. lost per week

DAILY CALORIE BALANCE:

Each week you should recalculate your **DAILY CALORIE BALANCE** based on your new weight.

* Remember, women should eat at least 1,200 calories per day and men should eat 1,500 to maintain a healthy diet.

FAT

Diet experts recommend consuming between 20% and 30% of your daily calories through fat. Each gram of fat contains nine calories, so if you figure out that you should be on a diet of 1,500 calories per day, then you should eat between 33 and 50 grams of fat per day.

To find the right **DAILY FAT BALANCE** for you, use the following formula:

DAILY CALORIE BALANCE x .25 (healthy percent of fat of calories from fat) ÷ 9 (calories in a gram of fat) = **DAILY FAT BALANCE** (in grams)

> DAILY FAT BALANCE:

Each week you should recalculate your Daily Fat Balance based on your new weight.

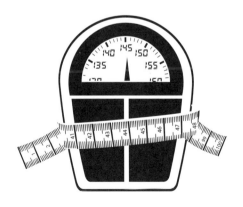

Personal Goals

(Use the extra pages if your first plan doesn't work for you.)

START DATE_____ END DATE_____

MY GOAL

_____

_____

_____

_____

_____

_____

_____

_____

MY PLAN

_____

_____

_____

_____

_____

_____

_____

_____

DAILY FOOD TARGETS

CALORIES	PROTEIN	CARBS	FAT	SODIUM	FIBER	# OF FRUITS & VEGETABLES

PHYSICAL ACTIVITY TARGETS

DAILY ACTIVITY	QUANTITY/TIME

WEEKLY ACTIVITY	QUANTITY/TIME

MY STATISTICS

GOAL	MEASUREMENTS	BEFORE	AFTER	NET GAIN OR LOSS
	WEIGHT			
	CHOLESTEROL LEVEL			
	BLOOD PRESSURE			
	CHEST			
	WAIST			
	HIPS			
	NECK			
	UPPER ARMS			
	THIGHS			
	CALVES			

Personal Goals

(Use the extra pages if your first plan doesn't work for you.)

START DATE_____   END DATE_____

MY GOAL

_____

_____

_____

_____

_____

_____

_____

_____

_____

_____

MY PLAN

_____

_____

_____

_____

_____

_____

_____

_____

_____

_____

DAILY FOOD TARGETS

CALORIES	PROTEIN	CARBS	FAT	SODIUM	FIBER	# OF FRUITS & VEGETABLES

PHYSICAL ACTIVITY TARGETS

DAILY ACTIVITY	QUANTITY/TIME

WEEKLY ACTIVITY	QUANTITY/TIME

MY STATISTICS

GOAL	MEASUREMENTS	BEFORE	AFTER	NET GAIN OR LOSS
	WEIGHT			
	CHOLESTEROL LEVEL			
	BLOOD PRESSURE			
	CHEST			
	WAIST			
	HIPS			
	NECK			
	UPPER ARMS			
	THIGHS			
	CALVES			

General Goals

Before & After

Use this space to document your success. Tape or paste photos showing the beginning and end of your personal health journey.

BEFORE

AFTER

Daily

DIET & EXERCISE

RECORDS

Your journal will be your quick-reference, easy-to-use, all-inclusive tracker. Use it to record the calories, protein, carbs, fat, sodium, and fiber in all the foods you eat. Keeping records will show you what foods are your favorites, which you find hard to resist, and what you need to cut from or add to your diet, as well as hold you accountable for everything you eat.

In addition to your diet, you will record all the exercise that you do and how many calories you burned doing it. You will also be tracking how much water you drink and how many fruits and vegetables you eat. Plus, there is a comments section where you can write down whatever you want for that day: where you went right or wrong, recipes or foods you come across that you love and love you back, or something that inspired you to stay on course.

The next two pages are from a sample journal. This sample dieter is a 5' 6" woman who started out at 182 pounds. Take a look at how she's doing on pages 22–23. After that, you'll be fully prepared to start your new healthy, feel-better, look-better life.

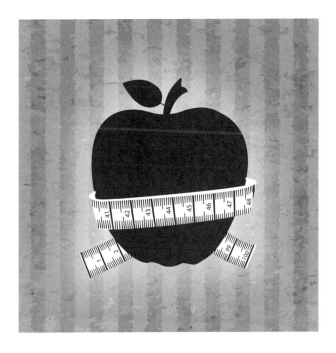

DATE Saturday, December 5			**WEEK #** 5		**DAY** 35			
CALORIE GOAL 1,580			FAT GOAL 44					

TIME	AMT	FOOD	CAL	PROTEIN	CARBS	FAT	SODIUM	FIBER
7:30am	8 oz	cranberry juice	144	–	34	–	5	–
	1 cup	coffee w/1 sugar	20	–	4	–	5	–
	2	eggs	132	12	–	8	124	–
1 pm	½	head of Boston lettuce	11	–	2	–	3	1
	1	tomato	38	2	7	1	9	2
	¼ cup	shredded cheddar	113	7	–	9	175	–
	2 tbs.	low-cal blue cheese dressing	30	1	–	2	277	–
	12 oz	diet soda	–	–	4	–	20	–
3 pm	3	chocolate chip cookies	144	1	16	6	96	–
6 pm	½	chicken breast	142	27	–	3	63	–
	1 tbs.	olive oil	119	–	–	14	–	–
	1	baked potato	220	5	63	–	17	4
	1 cup	string beans	44	2	10	–	6	3
	7 oz	white wine	140	–	5	–	1	–
7 pm	1 cup	vanilla ice cream	236	4	34	14	106	–
		TOTALS FOR TODAY	1,533	61	179	57	907	10

# of 8-ounce glasses of water drank today:

EXERCISE

TIME	TYPE	INTENSITY	DURATION	CAL BURNED
6:30pm	Stationary Bicycle	light	30 min.	240
	TOTALS FOR TODAY			

VITAMINS/SUPPLEMENTS/MEDS

DESCRIPTION	QUANTITY
multivitamin	1

DAILY WEIGH IN

ORIGINAL WEIGHT	NEW WEIGHT	WEIGHT CHANGE	POUNDS LEFT BEFORE GOAL
182	174	8	25

NOTES ABOUT TODAY

Feeling great! My favorite jeans are starting to fit again, and Sarah mentioned how great I look at lunch.

I was a little bit hungry this afternoon - I'll try to focus on getting in more water tomorrow and see if that helps.

DATE				WEEK #		DAY	

CALORIE GOAL				FAT GOAL			

TIME	AMT	FOOD	CAL	PROTEIN	CARBS	FAT	SODIUM	FIBER
		TOTALS FOR TODAY						

# of 8-ounce glasses of water drank today:

EXERCISE

TIME	TYPE	INTENSITY	DURATION	CAL BURNED
TOTALS FOR TODAY				

VITAMINS/SUPPLEMENTS/MEDS

DESCRIPTION	QUANTITY

DAILY WEIGH IN

ORIGINAL WEIGHT	NEW WEIGHT	WEIGHT CHANGE	POUNDS LEFT BEFORE GOAL

NOTES ABOUT TODAY

DATE			WEEK #	DAY

CALORIE GOAL	FAT GOAL

TIME	AMT	FOOD	CAL	PROTEIN	CARBS	FAT	SODIUM	FIBER
TOTALS FOR TODAY								

# of 8-ounce glasses of water drank today:

EXERCISE

TIME	TYPE	INTENSITY	DURATION	CAL BURNED
TOTALS FOR TODAY				

VITAMINS/SUPPLEMENTS/MEDS

DESCRIPTION	QUANTITY

DAILY WEIGH IN

ORIGINAL WEIGHT	NEW WEIGHT	WEIGHT CHANGE	POUNDS LEFT BEFORE GOAL

NOTES ABOUT TODAY

DAILY DIET & EXERCISE RECORDS

DATE | **WEEK #** | **DAY**

CALORIE GOAL | FAT GOAL

TIME	AMT	FOOD	CAL	PROTEIN	CARBS	FAT	SODIUM	FIBER
TOTALS FOR TODAY								

# of 8-ounce glasses of water drank today:

EXERCISE

TIME	TYPE	INTENSITY	DURATION	CAL BURNED
TOTALS FOR TODAY				

VITAMINS/SUPPLEMENTS/MEDS

DESCRIPTION	QUANTITY

DAILY WEIGH IN

ORIGINAL WEIGHT	NEW WEIGHT	WEIGHT CHANGE	POUNDS LEFT BEFORE GOAL

NOTES ABOUT TODAY

DATE		WEEK #	DAY

CALORIE GOAL	FAT GOAL

TIME	AMT	FOOD	CAL	PROTEIN	CARBS	FAT	SODIUM	FIBER
		TOTALS FOR TODAY						

# of 8-ounce glasses of water drank today:

EXERCISE

TIME	TYPE	INTENSITY	DURATION	CAL BURNED
	TOTALS FOR TODAY			

VITAMINS/SUPPLEMENTS/MEDS

DESCRIPTION	QUANTITY

DAILY WEIGH IN

ORIGINAL WEIGHT	NEW WEIGHT	WEIGHT CHANGE	POUNDS LEFT BEFORE GOAL

NOTES ABOUT TODAY

DAILY DIET & EXERCISE RECORDS

DATE		WEEK #	DAY

CALORIE GOAL	FAT GOAL

TIME	AMT	FOOD	CAL	PROTEIN	CARBS	FAT	SODIUM	FIBER
		TOTALS FOR TODAY						

# of 8-ounce glasses of water drank today:

EXERCISE

TIME	TYPE	INTENSITY	DURATION	CAL BURNED
	TOTALS FOR TODAY			

VITAMINS/SUPPLEMENTS/MEDS

DESCRIPTION	QUANTITY

DAILY WEIGH IN

ORIGINAL WEIGHT	NEW WEIGHT	WEIGHT CHANGE	POUNDS LEFT BEFORE GOAL

NOTES ABOUT TODAY

DATE				WEEK #		DAY			

CALORIE GOAL

FAT GOAL

TIME	AMT	FOOD	CAL	PROTEIN	CARBS	FAT	SODIUM	FIBER
TOTALS FOR TODAY								

# of 8-ounce glasses of water drank today:

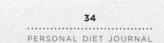

EXERCISE

TIME	TYPE	INTENSITY	DURATION	CAL BURNED
	TOTALS FOR TODAY			

VITAMINS/SUPPLEMENTS/MEDS

DESCRIPTION	QUANTITY

DAILY WEIGH IN

ORIGINAL WEIGHT	NEW WEIGHT	WEIGHT CHANGE	POUNDS LEFT BEFORE GOAL

NOTES ABOUT TODAY

DATE		WEEK #	DAY

CALORIE GOAL	FAT GOAL

TIME	AMT	FOOD	CAL	PROTEIN	CARBS	FAT	SODIUM	FIBER
TOTALS FOR TODAY								

# of 8-ounce glasses of water drank today:

EXERCISE

TIME	TYPE	INTENSITY	DURATION	CAL BURNED
TOTALS FOR TODAY				

VITAMINS/SUPPLEMENTS/MEDS

DESCRIPTION	QUANTITY

DAILY WEIGH IN

ORIGINAL WEIGHT	NEW WEIGHT	WEIGHT CHANGE	POUNDS LEFT BEFORE GOAL

NOTES ABOUT TODAY

DATE			WEEK #	DAY

CALORIE GOAL	FAT GOAL

TIME	AMT	FOOD	CAL	PROTEIN	CARBS	FAT	SODIUM	FIBER
TOTALS FOR TODAY								

# of 8-ounce glasses of water drank today:

EXERCISE

TIME	TYPE	INTENSITY	DURATION	CAL BURNED
TOTALS FOR TODAY				

VITAMINS/SUPPLEMENTS/MEDS

DESCRIPTION	QUANTITY

DAILY WEIGH IN

ORIGINAL WEIGHT	NEW WEIGHT	WEIGHT CHANGE	POUNDS LEFT BEFORE GOAL

NOTES ABOUT TODAY

DATE			WEEK #	DAY

CALORIE GOAL

FAT GOAL

TIME	AMT	FOOD	CAL	PROTEIN	CARBS	FAT	SODIUM	FIBER
	TOTALS FOR TODAY							

# of 8-ounce glasses of water drank today:

EXERCISE

TIME	TYPE	INTENSITY	DURATION	CAL BURNED
	TOTALS FOR TODAY			

VITAMINS/SUPPLEMENTS/MEDS

DESCRIPTION	QUANTITY

DAILY WEIGH IN

ORIGINAL WEIGHT	NEW WEIGHT	WEIGHT CHANGE	POUNDS LEFT BEFORE GOAL

NOTES ABOUT TODAY

DATE				WEEK #		DAY	

CALORIE GOAL

FAT GOAL

TIME	AMT	FOOD	CAL	PROTEIN	CARBS	FAT	SODIUM	FIBER
TOTALS FOR TODAY								

# of 8-ounce glasses of water drank today:

EXERCISE

TIME	TYPE	INTENSITY	DURATION	CAL BURNED
	TOTALS FOR TODAY			

VITAMINS/SUPPLEMENTS/MEDS

DESCRIPTION	QUANTITY

DAILY WEIGH IN

ORIGINAL WEIGHT	NEW WEIGHT	WEIGHT CHANGE	POUNDS LEFT BEFORE GOAL

NOTES ABOUT TODAY

DATE			WEEK #		DAY	

CALORIE GOAL		FAT GOAL	

TIME	AMT	FOOD	CAL	PROTEIN	CARBS	FAT	SODIUM	FIBER
TOTALS FOR TODAY								

# of 8-ounce glasses of water drank today:

EXERCISE

TIME	TYPE	INTENSITY	DURATION	CAL BURNED
TOTALS FOR TODAY				

VITAMINS/SUPPLEMENTS/MEDS

DESCRIPTION	QUANTITY

DAILY WEIGH IN

ORIGINAL WEIGHT	NEW WEIGHT	WEIGHT CHANGE	POUNDS LEFT BEFORE GOAL

NOTES ABOUT TODAY

DATE			WEEK #		DAY	

CALORIE GOAL		FAT GOAL	

TIME	AMT	FOOD	CAL	PROTEIN	CARBS	FAT	SODIUM	FIBER
	TOTALS FOR TODAY							

# of 8-ounce glasses of water drank today:

EXERCISE

TIME	TYPE	INTENSITY	DURATION	CAL BURNED
	TOTALS FOR TODAY			

VITAMINS/SUPPLEMENTS/MEDS

DESCRIPTION	QUANTITY

DAILY WEIGH IN

ORIGINAL WEIGHT	NEW WEIGHT	WEIGHT CHANGE	POUNDS LEFT BEFORE GOAL

NOTES ABOUT TODAY

DATE			WEEK #		DAY	

CALORIE GOAL			FAT GOAL			

TIME	AMT	FOOD	CAL	PROTEIN	CARBS	FAT	SODIUM	FIBER
TOTALS FOR TODAY								

# of 8-ounce glasses of water drank today:

EXERCISE

TIME	TYPE	INTENSITY	DURATION	CAL BURNED
	TOTALS FOR TODAY			

VITAMINS/SUPPLEMENTS/MEDS

DESCRIPTION	QUANTITY

DAILY WEIGH IN

ORIGINAL WEIGHT	NEW WEIGHT	WEIGHT CHANGE	POUNDS LEFT BEFORE GOAL

NOTES ABOUT TODAY

DAILY DIET & EXERCISE RECORDS

DATE			WEEK #		DAY	

CALORIE GOAL		FAT GOAL	

TIME	AMT	FOOD	CAL	PROTEIN	CARBS	FAT	SODIUM	FIBER
TOTALS FOR TODAY								

# of 8-ounce glasses of water drank today:

EXERCISE

TIME	TYPE	INTENSITY	DURATION	CAL BURNED
TOTALS FOR TODAY				

VITAMINS/SUPPLEMENTS/MEDS

DESCRIPTION	QUANTITY

DAILY WEIGH IN

ORIGINAL WEIGHT	NEW WEIGHT	WEIGHT CHANGE	POUNDS LEFT BEFORE GOAL

NOTES ABOUT TODAY

TIME	AMT	FOOD	CAL	PROTEIN	CARBS	FAT	SODIUM	FIBER
	TOTALS FOR TODAY							

# of 8-ounce glasses of water drank today:

EXERCISE

TIME	TYPE	INTENSITY	DURATION	CAL BURNED
	TOTALS FOR TODAY			

VITAMINS/SUPPLEMENTS/MEDS

DESCRIPTION	QUANTITY

DAILY WEIGH IN

ORIGINAL WEIGHT	NEW WEIGHT	WEIGHT CHANGE	POUNDS LEFT BEFORE GOAL

NOTES ABOUT TODAY

DAILY DIET & EXERCISE RECORDS

DATE			WEEK #		DAY	

CALORIE GOAL

FAT GOAL

TIME	AMT	FOOD	CAL	PROTEIN	CARBS	FAT	SODIUM	FIBER
	TOTALS FOR TODAY							

# of 8-ounce glasses of water drank today:

EXERCISE

TIME	TYPE	INTENSITY	DURATION	CAL BURNED
	TOTALS FOR TODAY			

VITAMINS/SUPPLEMENTS/MEDS

DESCRIPTION	QUANTITY

DAILY WEIGH IN

ORIGINAL WEIGHT	NEW WEIGHT	WEIGHT CHANGE	POUNDS LEFT BEFORE GOAL

NOTES ABOUT TODAY

DATE				WEEK #		DAY			

CALORIE GOAL

FAT GOAL

TIME	AMT	FOOD	CAL	PROTEIN	CARBS	FAT	SODIUM	FIBER
	TOTALS FOR TODAY							

# of 8-ounce glasses of water drank today:

EXERCISE

TIME	TYPE	INTENSITY	DURATION	CAL BURNED
	TOTALS FOR TODAY			

VITAMINS/SUPPLEMENTS/MEDS

DESCRIPTION	QUANTITY

DAILY WEIGH IN

ORIGINAL WEIGHT	NEW WEIGHT	WEIGHT CHANGE	POUNDS LEFT BEFORE GOAL

NOTES ABOUT TODAY

DATE					WEEK #		DAY		

CALORIE GOAL					FAT GOAL				

TIME	AMT	FOOD	CAL	PROTEIN	CARBS	FAT	SODIUM	FIBER
		TOTALS FOR TODAY						

# of 8-ounce glasses of water drank today:

EXERCISE

TIME	TYPE	INTENSITY	DURATION	CAL BURNED
	TOTALS FOR TODAY			

VITAMINS/SUPPLEMENTS/MEDS

DESCRIPTION	QUANTITY

DAILY WEIGH IN

ORIGINAL WEIGHT	NEW WEIGHT	WEIGHT CHANGE	POUNDS LEFT BEFORE GOAL

NOTES ABOUT TODAY

DATE		WEEK #		DAY

CALORIE GOAL	FAT GOAL

TIME	AMT	FOOD	CAL	PROTEIN	CARBS	FAT	SODIUM	FIBER
TOTALS FOR TODAY								

# of 8-ounce glasses of water drank today:

EXERCISE

TIME	TYPE	INTENSITY	DURATION	CAL BURNED
	TOTALS FOR TODAY			

VITAMINS/SUPPLEMENTS/MEDS

DESCRIPTION	QUANTITY

DAILY WEIGH IN

ORIGINAL WEIGHT	NEW WEIGHT	WEIGHT CHANGE	POUNDS LEFT BEFORE GOAL

NOTES ABOUT TODAY

DATE		WEEK #		DAY

CALORIE GOAL	FAT GOAL

TIME	AMT	FOOD	CAL	PROTEIN	CARBS	FAT	SODIUM	FIBER
	TOTALS FOR TODAY							

# of 8-ounce glasses of water drank today:

EXERCISE

TIME	TYPE	INTENSITY	DURATION	CAL BURNED
TOTALS FOR TODAY				

VITAMINS/SUPPLEMENTS/MEDS

DESCRIPTION	QUANTITY

DAILY WEIGH IN

ORIGINAL WEIGHT	NEW WEIGHT	WEIGHT CHANGE	POUNDS LEFT BEFORE GOAL

NOTES ABOUT TODAY

DATE			WEEK #	DAY
CALORIE GOAL			FAT GOAL	

TIME	AMT	FOOD	CAL	PROTEIN	CARBS	FAT	SODIUM	FIBER

TOTALS FOR TODAY

# of 8-ounce glasses of water drank today:

EXERCISE

TIME	TYPE	INTENSITY	DURATION	CAL BURNED
	TOTALS FOR TODAY			

VITAMINS/SUPPLEMENTS/MEDS

DESCRIPTION	QUANTITY

DAILY WEIGH IN

ORIGINAL WEIGHT	NEW WEIGHT	WEIGHT CHANGE	POUNDS LEFT BEFORE GOAL

NOTES ABOUT TODAY

DATE			WEEK #	DAY

CALORIE GOAL

FAT GOAL

TIME	AMT	FOOD	CAL	PROTEIN	CARBS	FAT	SODIUM	FIBER
	TOTALS FOR TODAY							

# of 8-ounce glasses of water drank today:

EXERCISE

TIME	TYPE	INTENSITY	DURATION	CAL BURNED
TOTALS FOR TODAY				

VITAMINS/SUPPLEMENTS/MEDS

DESCRIPTION	QUANTITY

DAILY WEIGH IN

ORIGINAL WEIGHT	NEW WEIGHT	WEIGHT CHANGE	POUNDS LEFT BEFORE GOAL

NOTES ABOUT TODAY

DATE			WEEK #	DAY

CALORIE GOAL	FAT GOAL

TIME	AMT	FOOD	CAL	PROTEIN	CARBS	FAT	SODIUM	FIBER
		TOTALS FOR TODAY						

# of 8-ounce glasses of water drank today:

EXERCISE

TIME	TYPE	INTENSITY	DURATION	CAL BURNED
	TOTALS FOR TODAY			

VITAMINS/SUPPLEMENTS/MEDS

DESCRIPTION	QUANTITY

DAILY WEIGH IN

ORIGINAL WEIGHT	NEW WEIGHT	WEIGHT CHANGE	POUNDS LEFT BEFORE GOAL

NOTES ABOUT TODAY

DATE		WEEK #	DAY

CALORIE GOAL	FAT GOAL

TIME	AMT	FOOD	CAL	PROTEIN	CARBS	FAT	SODIUM	FIBER
	TOTALS FOR TODAY							

# of 8-ounce glasses of water drank today:

EXERCISE

TIME	TYPE	INTENSITY	DURATION	CAL BURNED
	TOTALS FOR TODAY			

VITAMINS/SUPPLEMENTS/MEDS

DESCRIPTION	QUANTITY

DAILY WEIGH IN

ORIGINAL WEIGHT	NEW WEIGHT	WEIGHT CHANGE	POUNDS LEFT BEFORE GOAL

NOTES ABOUT TODAY

DATE				WEEK #		DAY	

CALORIE GOAL				FAT GOAL			

TIME	AMT	FOOD	CAL	PROTEIN	CARBS	FAT	SODIUM	FIBER
		TOTALS FOR TODAY						

# of 8-ounce glasses of water drank today:

EXERCISE

TIME	TYPE	INTENSITY	DURATION	CAL BURNED
	TOTALS FOR TODAY			

VITAMINS/SUPPLEMENTS/MEDS

DESCRIPTION	QUANTITY

DAILY WEIGH IN

ORIGINAL WEIGHT	NEW WEIGHT	WEIGHT CHANGE	POUNDS LEFT BEFORE GOAL

NOTES ABOUT TODAY

DATE			WEEK #		DAY	

CALORIE GOAL			FAT GOAL			

TIME	AMT	FOOD	CAL	PROTEIN	CARBS	FAT	SODIUM	FIBER
	TOTALS FOR TODAY							

# of 8-ounce glasses of water drank today:

EXERCISE

TIME	TYPE	INTENSITY	DURATION	CAL BURNED
TOTALS FOR TODAY				

VITAMINS/SUPPLEMENTS/MEDS

DESCRIPTION	QUANTITY

DAILY WEIGH IN

ORIGINAL WEIGHT	NEW WEIGHT	WEIGHT CHANGE	POUNDS LEFT BEFORE GOAL

NOTES ABOUT TODAY

DATE				WEEK #		DAY		

CALORIE GOAL				FAT GOAL				

TIME	AMT	FOOD	CAL	PROTEIN	CARBS	FAT	SODIUM	FIBER
TOTALS FOR TODAY								

# of 8-ounce glasses of water drank today:

EXERCISE

TIME	TYPE	INTENSITY	DURATION	CAL BURNED
	TOTALS FOR TODAY			

VITAMINS/SUPPLEMENTS/MEDS

DESCRIPTION	QUANTITY

DAILY WEIGH IN

ORIGINAL WEIGHT	NEW WEIGHT	WEIGHT CHANGE	POUNDS LEFT BEFORE GOAL

NOTES ABOUT TODAY

DATE				WEEK #		DAY		

CALORIE GOAL				FAT GOAL				

TIME	AMT	FOOD	CAL	PROTEIN	CARBS	FAT	SODIUM	FIBER
	TOTALS FOR TODAY							

# of 8-ounce glasses of water drank today:

EXERCISE

TIME	TYPE	INTENSITY	DURATION	CAL BURNED
TOTALS FOR TODAY			

VITAMINS/SUPPLEMENTS/MEDS

DESCRIPTION	QUANTITY

DAILY WEIGH IN

ORIGINAL WEIGHT	NEW WEIGHT	WEIGHT CHANGE	POUNDS LEFT BEFORE GOAL

NOTES ABOUT TODAY

DATE		WEEK #	DAY

CALORIE GOAL	FAT GOAL

TIME	AMT	FOOD	CAL	PROTEIN	CARBS	FAT	SODIUM	FIBER
		TOTALS FOR TODAY						

# of 8-ounce glasses of water drank today:

EXERCISE

TIME	TYPE	INTENSITY	DURATION	CAL BURNED
	TOTALS FOR TODAY			

VITAMINS/SUPPLEMENTS/MEDS

DESCRIPTION	QUANTITY

DAILY WEIGH IN

ORIGINAL WEIGHT	NEW WEIGHT	WEIGHT CHANGE	POUNDS LEFT BEFORE GOAL

NOTES ABOUT TODAY

DATE				WEEK #		DAY			

CALORIE GOAL				FAT GOAL					

TIME	AMT	FOOD	CAL	PROTEIN	CARBS	FAT	SODIUM	FIBER
		TOTALS FOR TODAY						

# of 8-ounce glasses of water drank today:

EXERCISE

TIME	TYPE	INTENSITY	DURATION	CAL BURNED
	TOTALS FOR TODAY			

VITAMINS/SUPPLEMENTS/MEDS

DESCRIPTION	QUANTITY

DAILY WEIGH IN

ORIGINAL WEIGHT	NEW WEIGHT	WEIGHT CHANGE	POUNDS LEFT BEFORE GOAL

NOTES ABOUT TODAY

DATE			WEEK #	DAY

CALORIE GOAL	FAT GOAL

TIME	AMT	FOOD	CAL	PROTEIN	CARBS	FAT	SODIUM	FIBER
TOTALS FOR TODAY								

# of 8-ounce glasses of water drank today:

EXERCISE

TIME	TYPE	INTENSITY	DURATION	CAL BURNED
	TOTALS FOR TODAY			

VITAMINS/SUPPLEMENTS/MEDS

DESCRIPTION	QUANTITY

DAILY WEIGH IN

ORIGINAL WEIGHT	NEW WEIGHT	WEIGHT CHANGE	POUNDS LEFT BEFORE GOAL

NOTES ABOUT TODAY

DATE			WEEK #		DAY	

CALORIE GOAL		FAT GOAL	

TIME	AMT	FOOD	CAL	PROTEIN	CARBS	FAT	SODIUM	FIBER
	TOTALS FOR TODAY							

# of 8-ounce glasses of water drank today:

EXERCISE

TIME	TYPE	INTENSITY	DURATION	CAL BURNED
	TOTALS FOR TODAY			

VITAMINS/SUPPLEMENTS/MEDS

DESCRIPTION	QUANTITY

DAILY WEIGH IN

ORIGINAL WEIGHT	NEW WEIGHT	WEIGHT CHANGE	POUNDS LEFT BEFORE GOAL

NOTES ABOUT TODAY

DAILY DIET & EXERCISE RECORDS

DATE			WEEK #	DAY
CALORIE GOAL			FAT GOAL	

TIME	AMT	FOOD	CAL	PROTEIN	CARBS	FAT	SODIUM	FIBER
		TOTALS FOR TODAY						

# of 8-ounce glasses of water drank today:

EXERCISE

TIME	TYPE	INTENSITY	DURATION	CAL BURNED
	TOTALS FOR TODAY			

VITAMINS/SUPPLEMENTS/MEDS

DESCRIPTION	QUANTITY

DAILY WEIGH IN

ORIGINAL WEIGHT	NEW WEIGHT	WEIGHT CHANGE	POUNDS LEFT BEFORE GOAL

NOTES ABOUT TODAY

DAILY DIET & EXERCISE RECORDS

DATE			WEEK #		DAY	
CALORIE GOAL			FAT GOAL			

TIME	AMT	FOOD	CAL	PROTEIN	CARBS	FAT	SODIUM	FIBER
	TOTALS FOR TODAY							

# of 8-ounce glasses of water drank today:

EXERCISE

TIME	TYPE	INTENSITY	DURATION	CAL BURNED
TOTALS FOR TODAY				

VITAMINS/SUPPLEMENTS/MEDS

DESCRIPTION	QUANTITY

DAILY WEIGH IN

ORIGINAL WEIGHT	NEW WEIGHT	WEIGHT CHANGE	POUNDS LEFT BEFORE GOAL

NOTES ABOUT TODAY

DAILY DIET & EXERCISE RECORDS

DATE			WEEK #	DAY

CALORIE GOAL	FAT GOAL

TIME	AMT	FOOD	CAL	PROTEIN	CARBS	FAT	SODIUM	FIBER
	TOTALS FOR TODAY							

# of 8-ounce glasses of water drank today:

EXERCISE

TIME	TYPE	INTENSITY	DURATION	CAL BURNED
TOTALS FOR TODAY				

VITAMINS/SUPPLEMENTS/MEDS

DESCRIPTION	QUANTITY

DAILY WEIGH IN

ORIGINAL WEIGHT	NEW WEIGHT	WEIGHT CHANGE	POUNDS LEFT BEFORE GOAL

NOTES ABOUT TODAY

DATE		WEEK #	DAY

CALORIE GOAL

FAT GOAL

TIME	AMT	FOOD	CAL	PROTEIN	CARBS	FAT	SODIUM	FIBER
	TOTALS FOR TODAY							

# of 8-ounce glasses of water drank today:

EXERCISE

TIME	TYPE	INTENSITY	DURATION	CAL BURNED
	TOTALS FOR TODAY			

VITAMINS/SUPPLEMENTS/MEDS

DESCRIPTION	QUANTITY

DAILY WEIGH IN

ORIGINAL WEIGHT	NEW WEIGHT	WEIGHT CHANGE	POUNDS LEFT BEFORE GOAL

NOTES ABOUT TODAY

DATE		WEEK #	DAY

CALORIE GOAL

FAT GOAL

TIME	AMT	FOOD	CAL	PROTEIN	CARBS	FAT	SODIUM	FIBER
		TOTALS FOR TODAY						

# of 8-ounce glasses of water drank today:

EXERCISE

TIME	TYPE	INTENSITY	DURATION	CAL BURNED
TOTALS FOR TODAY				

VITAMINS/SUPPLEMENTS/MEDS

DESCRIPTION	QUANTITY

DAILY WEIGH IN

ORIGINAL WEIGHT	NEW WEIGHT	WEIGHT CHANGE	POUNDS LEFT BEFORE GOAL

NOTES ABOUT TODAY

DATE		WEEK #	DAY

CALORIE GOAL	FAT GOAL

TIME	AMT	FOOD	CAL	PROTEIN	CARBS	FAT	SODIUM	FIBER
	TOTALS FOR TODAY							

# of 8-ounce glasses of water drank today:

EXERCISE

TIME	TYPE	INTENSITY	DURATION	CAL BURNED
TOTALS FOR TODAY				

VITAMINS/SUPPLEMENTS/MEDS

DESCRIPTION	QUANTITY

DAILY WEIGH IN

ORIGINAL WEIGHT	NEW WEIGHT	WEIGHT CHANGE	POUNDS LEFT BEFORE GOAL

NOTES ABOUT TODAY

DATE		WEEK #	DAY

CALORIE GOAL	FAT GOAL

TIME	AMT	FOOD	CAL	PROTEIN	CARBS	FAT	SODIUM	FIBER
		TOTALS FOR TODAY						

of 8-ounce glasses of water drank today:

EXERCISE

TIME	TYPE	INTENSITY	DURATION	CAL BURNED
	TOTALS FOR TODAY			

VITAMINS/SUPPLEMENTS/MEDS

DESCRIPTION	QUANTITY

DAILY WEIGH IN

ORIGINAL WEIGHT	NEW WEIGHT	WEIGHT CHANGE	POUNDS LEFT BEFORE GOAL

NOTES ABOUT TODAY

DATE					WEEK #		DAY		

CALORIE GOAL

FAT GOAL

TIME	AMT	FOOD	CAL	PROTEIN	CARBS	FAT	SODIUM	FIBER
	TOTALS FOR TODAY							

# of 8-ounce glasses of water drank today:

EXERCISE

TIME	TYPE	INTENSITY	DURATION	CAL BURNED
TOTALS FOR TODAY				

VITAMINS/SUPPLEMENTS/MEDS

DESCRIPTION	QUANTITY

DAILY WEIGH IN

ORIGINAL WEIGHT	NEW WEIGHT	WEIGHT CHANGE	POUNDS LEFT BEFORE GOAL

NOTES ABOUT TODAY

DATE		WEEK #	DAY

CALORIE GOAL	FAT GOAL

TIME	AMT	FOOD	CAL	PROTEIN	CARBS	FAT	SODIUM	FIBER
		TOTALS FOR TODAY						

# of 8-ounce glasses of water drank today:

EXERCISE

TIME	TYPE	INTENSITY	DURATION	CAL BURNED
	TOTALS FOR TODAY			

VITAMINS/SUPPLEMENTS/MEDS

DESCRIPTION	QUANTITY

DAILY WEIGH IN

ORIGINAL WEIGHT	NEW WEIGHT	WEIGHT CHANGE	POUNDS LEFT BEFORE GOAL

NOTES ABOUT TODAY

DAILY DIET & EXERCISE RECORDS

DATE				WEEK #		DAY			

CALORIE GOAL

FAT GOAL

TIME	AMT	FOOD	CAL	PROTEIN	CARBS	FAT	SODIUM	FIBER
	TOTALS FOR TODAY							

# of 8-ounce glasses of water drank today:

EXERCISE

TIME	TYPE	INTENSITY	DURATION	CAL BURNED
	TOTALS FOR TODAY			

VITAMINS/SUPPLEMENTS/MEDS

DESCRIPTION	QUANTITY

DAILY WEIGH IN

ORIGINAL WEIGHT	NEW WEIGHT	WEIGHT CHANGE	POUNDS LEFT BEFORE GOAL

NOTES ABOUT TODAY

DATE			WEEK #	DAY

CALORIE GOAL

FAT GOAL

TIME	AMT	FOOD	CAL	PROTEIN	CARBS	FAT	SODIUM	FIBER
	TOTALS FOR TODAY							

# of 8-ounce glasses of water drank today:

EXERCISE

TIME	TYPE	INTENSITY	DURATION	CAL BURNED
TOTALS FOR TODAY				

VITAMINS/SUPPLEMENTS/MEDS

DESCRIPTION	QUANTITY

DAILY WEIGH IN

ORIGINAL WEIGHT	NEW WEIGHT	WEIGHT CHANGE	POUNDS LEFT BEFORE GOAL

NOTES ABOUT TODAY

DATE			WEEK #	DAY

CALORIE GOAL	FAT GOAL

TIME	AMT	FOOD	CAL	PROTEIN	CARBS	FAT	SODIUM	FIBER
	TOTALS FOR TODAY							

# of 8-ounce glasses of water drank today:

EXERCISE

TIME	TYPE	INTENSITY	DURATION	CAL BURNED
TOTALS FOR TODAY				

VITAMINS/SUPPLEMENTS/MEDS

DESCRIPTION	QUANTITY

DAILY WEIGH IN

ORIGINAL WEIGHT	NEW WEIGHT	WEIGHT CHANGE	POUNDS LEFT BEFORE GOAL

NOTES ABOUT TODAY

DATE				WEEK #		DAY			
CALORIE GOAL					FAT GOAL				

TIME	AMT	FOOD	CAL	PROTEIN	CARBS	FAT	SODIUM	FIBER
	TOTALS FOR TODAY							

# of 8-ounce glasses of water drank today:

EXERCISE

TIME	TYPE	INTENSITY	DURATION	CAL BURNED
	TOTALS FOR TODAY			

VITAMINS/SUPPLEMENTS/MEDS

DESCRIPTION	QUANTITY

DAILY WEIGH IN

ORIGINAL WEIGHT	NEW WEIGHT	WEIGHT CHANGE	POUNDS LEFT BEFORE GOAL

NOTES ABOUT TODAY

DAILY DIET & EXERCISE RECORDS

DATE		WEEK #	DAY

CALORIE GOAL	FAT GOAL

TIME	AMT	FOOD	CAL	PROTEIN	CARBS	FAT	SODIUM	FIBER
	TOTALS FOR TODAY							

# of 8-ounce glasses of water drank today:

EXERCISE

TIME	TYPE	INTENSITY	DURATION	CAL BURNED
TOTALS FOR TODAY				

VITAMINS/SUPPLEMENTS/MEDS

DESCRIPTION	QUANTITY

DAILY WEIGH IN

ORIGINAL WEIGHT	NEW WEIGHT	WEIGHT CHANGE	POUNDS LEFT BEFORE GOAL

NOTES ABOUT TODAY

DATE			WEEK #	DAY

CALORIE GOAL	FAT GOAL

TIME	AMT	FOOD	CAL	PROTEIN	CARBS	FAT	SODIUM	FIBER
	TOTALS FOR TODAY							

# of 8-ounce glasses of water drank today:

EXERCISE

TIME	TYPE	INTENSITY	DURATION	CAL BURNED
	TOTALS FOR TODAY			

VITAMINS/SUPPLEMENTS/MEDS

DESCRIPTION	QUANTITY

DAILY WEIGH IN

ORIGINAL WEIGHT	NEW WEIGHT	WEIGHT CHANGE	POUNDS LEFT BEFORE GOAL

NOTES ABOUT TODAY

DATE			WEEK #		DAY	

CALORIE GOAL	FAT GOAL

TIME	AMT	FOOD	CAL	PROTEIN	CARBS	FAT	SODIUM	FIBER
TOTALS FOR TODAY								

# of 8-ounce glasses of water drank today:

EXERCISE

TIME	TYPE	INTENSITY	DURATION	CAL BURNED
TOTALS FOR TODAY				

VITAMINS/SUPPLEMENTS/MEDS

DESCRIPTION	QUANTITY

DAILY WEIGH IN

ORIGINAL WEIGHT	NEW WEIGHT	WEIGHT CHANGE	POUNDS LEFT BEFORE GOAL

NOTES ABOUT TODAY

DATE				WEEK #		DAY	

CALORIE GOAL				FAT GOAL			

TIME	AMT	FOOD	CAL	PROTEIN	CARBS	FAT	SODIUM	FIBER
	TOTALS FOR TODAY							

# of 8-ounce glasses of water drank today:

EXERCISE

TIME	TYPE	INTENSITY	DURATION	CAL BURNED
TOTALS FOR TODAY				

VITAMINS/SUPPLEMENTS/MEDS

DESCRIPTION	QUANTITY

DAILY WEIGH IN

ORIGINAL WEIGHT	NEW WEIGHT	WEIGHT CHANGE	POUNDS LEFT BEFORE GOAL

NOTES ABOUT TODAY

DATE		WEEK #		DAY

CALORIE GOAL

FAT GOAL

TIME	AMT	FOOD	CAL	PROTEIN	CARBS	FAT	SODIUM	FIBER
TOTALS FOR TODAY								

# of 8-ounce glasses of water drank today:

EXERCISE

TIME	TYPE	INTENSITY	DURATION	CAL BURNED
TOTALS FOR TODAY				

VITAMINS/SUPPLEMENTS/MEDS

DESCRIPTION	QUANTITY

DAILY WEIGH IN

ORIGINAL WEIGHT	NEW WEIGHT	WEIGHT CHANGE	POUNDS LEFT BEFORE GOAL

NOTES ABOUT TODAY

DATE			WEEK #	DAY

CALORIE GOAL

FAT GOAL

TIME	AMT	FOOD	CAL	PROTEIN	CARBS	FAT	SODIUM	FIBER
TOTALS FOR TODAY								

# of 8-ounce glasses of water drank today:

EXERCISE

TIME	TYPE	INTENSITY	DURATION	CAL BURNED
	TOTALS FOR TODAY			

VITAMINS/SUPPLEMENTS/MEDS

DESCRIPTION	QUANTITY

DAILY WEIGH IN

ORIGINAL WEIGHT	NEW WEIGHT	WEIGHT CHANGE	POUNDS LEFT BEFORE GOAL

NOTES ABOUT TODAY

DATE		WEEK #	DAY

CALORIE GOAL	FAT GOAL

TIME	AMT	FOOD	CAL	PROTEIN	CARBS	FAT	SODIUM	FIBER
		TOTALS FOR TODAY						

# of 8-ounce glasses of water drank today:

EXERCISE

TIME	TYPE	INTENSITY	DURATION	CAL BURNED
	TOTALS FOR TODAY			

VITAMINS/SUPPLEMENTS/MEDS

DESCRIPTION	QUANTITY

DAILY WEIGH IN

ORIGINAL WEIGHT	NEW WEIGHT	WEIGHT CHANGE	POUNDS LEFT BEFORE GOAL

NOTES ABOUT TODAY

DATE		WEEK #		DAY	

CALORIE GOAL	FAT GOAL

TIME	AMT	FOOD	CAL	PROTEIN	CARBS	FAT	SODIUM	FIBER
	TOTALS FOR TODAY							

# of 8-ounce glasses of water drank today:

EXERCISE

TIME	TYPE	INTENSITY	DURATION	CAL BURNED
	TOTALS FOR TODAY			

VITAMINS/SUPPLEMENTS/MEDS

DESCRIPTION	QUANTITY

DAILY WEIGH IN

ORIGINAL WEIGHT	NEW WEIGHT	WEIGHT CHANGE	POUNDS LEFT BEFORE GOAL

NOTES ABOUT TODAY

DAILY DIET & EXERCISE RECORDS

DATE		WEEK #		DAY	

CALORIE GOAL		FAT GOAL	

TIME	AMT	FOOD	CAL	PROTEIN	CARBS	FAT	SODIUM	FIBER
		TOTALS FOR TODAY						

# of 8-ounce glasses of water drank today:

EXERCISE

TIME	TYPE	INTENSITY	DURATION	CAL BURNED
	TOTALS FOR TODAY			

VITAMINS/SUPPLEMENTS/MEDS

DESCRIPTION	QUANTITY

DAILY WEIGH IN

ORIGINAL WEIGHT	NEW WEIGHT	WEIGHT CHANGE	POUNDS LEFT BEFORE GOAL

NOTES ABOUT TODAY

DATE			WEEK #		DAY	

CALORIE GOAL	FAT GOAL

TIME	AMT	FOOD	CAL	PROTEIN	CARBS	FAT	SODIUM	FIBER
		TOTALS FOR TODAY						

# of 8-ounce glasses of water drank today:

EXERCISE

TIME	TYPE	INTENSITY	DURATION	CAL BURNED
	TOTALS FOR TODAY			

VITAMINS/SUPPLEMENTS/MEDS

DESCRIPTION	QUANTITY

DAILY WEIGH IN

ORIGINAL WEIGHT	NEW WEIGHT	WEIGHT CHANGE	POUNDS LEFT BEFORE GOAL

NOTES ABOUT TODAY

DATE		WEEK #	DAY

CALORIE GOAL	FAT GOAL

TIME	AMT	FOOD	CAL	PROTEIN	CARBS	FAT	SODIUM	FIBER
	TOTALS FOR TODAY							

# of 8-ounce glasses of water drank today:

EXERCISE

TIME	TYPE	INTENSITY	DURATION	CAL BURNED
	TOTALS FOR TODAY			

VITAMINS/SUPPLEMENTS/MEDS

DESCRIPTION	QUANTITY

DAILY WEIGH IN

ORIGINAL WEIGHT	NEW WEIGHT	WEIGHT CHANGE	POUNDS LEFT BEFORE GOAL

NOTES ABOUT TODAY

DATE				WEEK #		DAY	

CALORIE GOAL		FAT GOAL	

TIME	AMT	FOOD	CAL	PROTEIN	CARBS	FAT	SODIUM	FIBER
TOTALS FOR TODAY								

# of 8-ounce glasses of water drank today:

EXERCISE

TIME	TYPE	INTENSITY	DURATION	CAL BURNED
TOTALS FOR TODAY				

VITAMINS/SUPPLEMENTS/MEDS

DESCRIPTION	QUANTITY

DAILY WEIGH IN

ORIGINAL WEIGHT	NEW WEIGHT	WEIGHT CHANGE	POUNDS LEFT BEFORE GOAL

NOTES ABOUT TODAY

		DATE				WEEK #		DAY	

CALORIE GOAL					FAT GOAL				

TIME	AMT	FOOD	CAL	PROTEIN	CARBS	FAT	SODIUM	FIBER
	TOTALS FOR TODAY							

# of 8-ounce glasses of water drank today:

EXERCISE

TIME	TYPE	INTENSITY	DURATION	CAL BURNED
	TOTALS FOR TODAY			

VITAMINS/SUPPLEMENTS/MEDS

DESCRIPTION	QUANTITY

DAILY WEIGH IN

ORIGINAL WEIGHT	NEW WEIGHT	WEIGHT CHANGE	POUNDS LEFT BEFORE GOAL

NOTES ABOUT TODAY

DATE					WEEK #		DAY	

CALORIE GOAL	FAT GOAL

TIME	AMT	FOOD	CAL	PROTEIN	CARBS	FAT	SODIUM	FIBER
	TOTALS FOR TODAY							

# of 8-ounce glasses of water drank today:

EXERCISE

TIME	TYPE	INTENSITY	DURATION	CAL BURNED
TOTALS FOR TODAY				

VITAMINS/SUPPLEMENTS/MEDS

DESCRIPTION	QUANTITY

DAILY WEIGH IN

ORIGINAL WEIGHT	NEW WEIGHT	WEIGHT CHANGE	POUNDS LEFT BEFORE GOAL

NOTES ABOUT TODAY

DATE		WEEK #	DAY

CALORIE GOAL	FAT GOAL

TIME	AMT	FOOD	CAL	PROTEIN	CARBS	FAT	SODIUM	FIBER
TOTALS FOR TODAY								

# of 8-ounce glasses of water drank today:

EXERCISE

TIME	TYPE	INTENSITY	DURATION	CAL BURNED
TOTALS FOR TODAY				

VITAMINS/SUPPLEMENTS/MEDS

DESCRIPTION	QUANTITY

DAILY WEIGH IN

ORIGINAL WEIGHT	NEW WEIGHT	WEIGHT CHANGE	POUNDS LEFT BEFORE GOAL

NOTES ABOUT TODAY

			DATE		WEEK #		DAY	

			CALORIE GOAL		FAT GOAL			

TIME	AMT	FOOD	CAL	PROTEIN	CARBS	FAT	SODIUM	FIBER
	TOTALS FOR TODAY							

of 8-ounce glasses of water drank today:

EXERCISE

TIME	TYPE	INTENSITY	DURATION	CAL BURNED
	TOTALS FOR TODAY			

VITAMINS/SUPPLEMENTS/MEDS

DESCRIPTION	QUANTITY

DAILY WEIGH IN

ORIGINAL WEIGHT	NEW WEIGHT	WEIGHT CHANGE	POUNDS LEFT BEFORE GOAL

NOTES ABOUT TODAY

DATE			WEEK #	DAY

CALORIE GOAL	FAT GOAL

TIME	AMT	FOOD	CAL	PROTEIN	CARBS	FAT	SODIUM	FIBER
	TOTALS FOR TODAY							

# of 8-ounce glasses of water drank today:

EXERCISE

TIME	TYPE	INTENSITY	DURATION	CAL BURNED
TOTALS FOR TODAY				

VITAMINS/SUPPLEMENTS/MEDS

DESCRIPTION	QUANTITY

DAILY WEIGH IN

ORIGINAL WEIGHT	NEW WEIGHT	WEIGHT CHANGE	POUNDS LEFT BEFORE GOAL

NOTES ABOUT TODAY

DATE				WEEK #		DAY			

CALORIE GOAL				FAT GOAL					

TIME	AMT	FOOD	CAL	PROTEIN	CARBS	FAT	SODIUM	FIBER
		TOTALS FOR TODAY						

# of 8-ounce glasses of water drank today:

EXERCISE

TIME	TYPE	INTENSITY	DURATION	CAL BURNED
	TOTALS FOR TODAY			

VITAMINS/SUPPLEMENTS/MEDS

DESCRIPTION	QUANTITY

DAILY WEIGH IN

ORIGINAL WEIGHT	NEW WEIGHT	WEIGHT CHANGE	POUNDS LEFT BEFORE GOAL

NOTES ABOUT TODAY

DATE		WEEK #	DAY

CALORIE GOAL	FAT GOAL

TIME	AMT	FOOD	CAL	PROTEIN	CARBS	FAT	SODIUM	FIBER
	TOTALS FOR TODAY							

# of 8-ounce glasses of water drank today:

EXERCISE

TIME	TYPE	INTENSITY	DURATION	CAL BURNED
	TOTALS FOR TODAY			

VITAMINS/SUPPLEMENTS/MEDS

DESCRIPTION	QUANTITY

DAILY WEIGH IN

ORIGINAL WEIGHT	NEW WEIGHT	WEIGHT CHANGE	POUNDS LEFT BEFORE GOAL

NOTES ABOUT TODAY

DATE			WEEK #	DAY

CALORIE GOAL	FAT GOAL

TIME	AMT	FOOD	CAL	PROTEIN	CARBS	FAT	SODIUM	FIBER
	TOTALS FOR TODAY							

# of 8-ounce glasses of water drank today:

EXERCISE

TIME	TYPE	INTENSITY	DURATION	CAL BURNED
TOTALS FOR TODAY				

VITAMINS/SUPPLEMENTS/MEDS

DESCRIPTION	QUANTITY

DAILY WEIGH IN

ORIGINAL WEIGHT	NEW WEIGHT	WEIGHT CHANGE	POUNDS LEFT BEFORE GOAL

NOTES ABOUT TODAY

DATE		WEEK #	DAY
CALORIE GOAL		FAT GOAL	

TIME	AMT	FOOD	CAL	PROTEIN	CARBS	FAT	SODIUM	FIBER
		TOTALS FOR TODAY						

# of 8-ounce glasses of water drank today:

EXERCISE

TIME	TYPE	INTENSITY	DURATION	CAL BURNED
	TOTALS FOR TODAY			

VITAMINS/SUPPLEMENTS/MEDS

DESCRIPTION	QUANTITY

DAILY WEIGH IN

ORIGINAL WEIGHT	NEW WEIGHT	WEIGHT CHANGE	POUNDS LEFT BEFORE GOAL

NOTES ABOUT TODAY

DATE			WEEK #		DAY				
CALORIE GOAL				FAT GOAL					

TIME	AMT	FOOD	CAL	PROTEIN	CARBS	FAT	SODIUM	FIBER
		TOTALS FOR TODAY						

# of 8-ounce glasses of water drank today:

EXERCISE

TIME	TYPE	INTENSITY	DURATION	CAL BURNED
TOTALS FOR TODAY				

VITAMINS/SUPPLEMENTS/MEDS

DESCRIPTION	QUANTITY

DAILY WEIGH IN

ORIGINAL WEIGHT	NEW WEIGHT	WEIGHT CHANGE	POUNDS LEFT BEFORE GOAL

NOTES ABOUT TODAY

DATE			WEEK #	DAY

CALORIE GOAL	FAT GOAL

TIME	AMT	FOOD	CAL	PROTEIN	CARBS	FAT	SODIUM	FIBER
	TOTALS FOR TODAY							

# of 8-ounce glasses of water drank today:

EXERCISE

TIME	TYPE	INTENSITY	DURATION	CAL BURNED
	TOTALS FOR TODAY			

VITAMINS/SUPPLEMENTS/MEDS

DESCRIPTION	QUANTITY

DAILY WEIGH IN

ORIGINAL WEIGHT	NEW WEIGHT	WEIGHT CHANGE	POUNDS LEFT BEFORE GOAL

NOTES ABOUT TODAY

DAILY DIET & EXERCISE RECORDS

DATE				WEEK #		DAY		

CALORIE GOAL	FAT GOAL

TIME	AMT	FOOD	CAL	PROTEIN	CARBS	FAT	SODIUM	FIBER

TOTALS FOR TODAY

# of 8-ounce glasses of water drank today:

EXERCISE

TIME	TYPE	INTENSITY	DURATION	CAL BURNED
TOTALS FOR TODAY				

VITAMINS/SUPPLEMENTS/MEDS

DESCRIPTION	QUANTITY

DAILY WEIGH IN

ORIGINAL WEIGHT	NEW WEIGHT	WEIGHT CHANGE	POUNDS LEFT BEFORE GOAL

NOTES ABOUT TODAY

DATE			WEEK #		DAY	

CALORIE GOAL	FAT GOAL

TIME	AMT	FOOD	CAL	PROTEIN	CARBS	FAT	SODIUM	FIBER
	TOTALS FOR TODAY							

# of 8-ounce glasses of water drank today:

EXERCISE

TIME	TYPE	INTENSITY	DURATION	CAL BURNED
TOTALS FOR TODAY				

VITAMINS/SUPPLEMENTS/MEDS

DESCRIPTION	QUANTITY

DAILY WEIGH IN

ORIGINAL WEIGHT	NEW WEIGHT	WEIGHT CHANGE	POUNDS LEFT BEFORE GOAL

NOTES ABOUT TODAY

	DATE		WEEK #	DAY

			CALORIE GOAL				FAT GOAL	

TIME	AMT	FOOD	CAL	PROTEIN	CARBS	FAT	SODIUM	FIBER
	TOTALS FOR TODAY							

# of 8-ounce glasses of water drank today:

EXERCISE

TIME	TYPE	INTENSITY	DURATION	CAL BURNED
TOTALS FOR TODAY				

VITAMINS/SUPPLEMENTS/MEDS

DESCRIPTION	QUANTITY

DAILY WEIGH IN

ORIGINAL WEIGHT	NEW WEIGHT	WEIGHT CHANGE	POUNDS LEFT BEFORE GOAL

NOTES ABOUT TODAY

DATE		WEEK #	DAY

CALORIE GOAL	FAT GOAL

TIME	AMT	FOOD	CAL	PROTEIN	CARBS	FAT	SODIUM	FIBER
		TOTALS FOR TODAY						

# of 8-ounce glasses of water drank today:

EXERCISE

TIME	TYPE	INTENSITY	DURATION	CAL BURNED
TOTALS FOR TODAY				

VITAMINS/SUPPLEMENTS/MEDS

DESCRIPTION	QUANTITY

DAILY WEIGH IN

ORIGINAL WEIGHT	NEW WEIGHT	WEIGHT CHANGE	POUNDS LEFT BEFORE GOAL

NOTES ABOUT TODAY

My
WEEKLY
PROGRESS

Weekly Statistics

Here, you can track your progress by recording statistics such as weight, blood pressure, waist circumference, average calorie intake, and physical activity for each week. Consult the totals from your **DAILY DIET & EXERCISE RECORDS,** and record whatever statistics you wish to track in the following tables. Additional spaces are provided after the suggested measurements, in case you would like to track other variables, such as the number of fast food meals you ate, or how many pints of beer you drank that week. In the chart below, our sample dieter has made some modest positive progress over the first two weeks in all but a few measurements.

MEASURMENTS	WEEK 1	WEEK 2	WEEK 3	WEEK 4	WEEK 5
WEIGHT	182	179			
BMI (SEE PAGE XX)	29.5	29			
CHOLESTEROL LEVEL					
BLOOD PRESSURE					
CHEST (INCHES)	35	35			
WAIST (INCHES)	32	31.5			
HIPS (INCHES)	39	39			
THIGHS (INCHES)					
UPPER ARMS (INCHES)					
AVG DAILY CALORIES	2100	1723			
AVG DAILY FAT	59	50			
AVG DAILY PROTEIN					
AVG DAILY CARBS	225	243			
GLASSES OF WATER	21	28			
# OF FRUITS & VEG					
HOURS OF EXERCISE	5	6			
CALORIES BURNED					
Dunkin Donuts Lattes	3	1			
Glasses of wine	4	3			
Miles run	10	11.25			

MEASURMENTS	WEEK 1	WEEK 2	WEEK 3	WEEK 4	WEEK 5
WEIGHT					
BMI (SEE PAGE 10)					
CHOLESTEROL LEVEL					
BLOOD PRESSURE					
CHEST (INCHES)					
WAIST (INCHES)					
HIPS (INCHES)					
THIGHS (INCHES)					
UPPER ARMS (INCHES)					
AVG DAILY CALORIES					
AVG DAILY FAT					
AVG DAILY PROTEIN					
AVG DAILY CARBS					
GLASSES OF WATER					
# OF FRUITS & VEG					
HOURS OF EXERCISE					
CALORIES BURNED					

MEASURMENTS	WEEK 6	WEEK 7	WEEK 8	WEEK 9	WEEK 10
WEIGHT					
BMI (SEE PAGE 10)					
CHOLESTEROL LEVEL					
BLOOD PRESSURE					
CHEST (INCHES)					
WAIST (INCHES)					
HIPS (INCHES)					
THIGHS (INCHES)					
UPPER ARMS (INCHES)					
AVG DAILY CALORIES					
AVG DAILY FAT					
AVG DAILY PROTEIN					
AVG DAILY CARBS					
GLASSES OF WATER					
# OF FRUITS & VEG					
HOURS OF EXERCISE					
CALORIES BURNED					

WEEKLY STATISTICS

Visualizing My Progress

As they say, a picture is worth a thousand words! The following graphs allow you to track your weekly progress visually. Take any statistics from your **WEEKLY STATISTICS** tables and plot them on the graphs on the following pages. You can even use the same graph to plot two different groups of data, as our sample dieter did in the graphs below, for easy comparison.

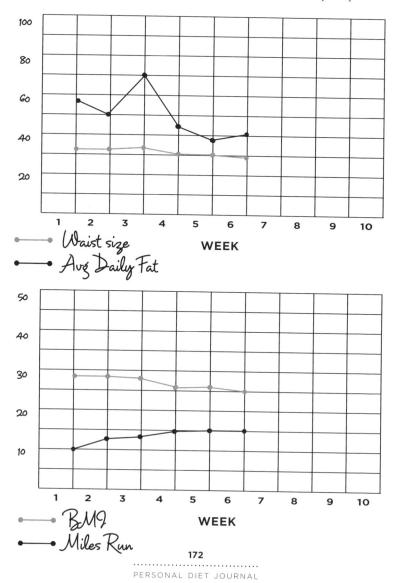

— Waist size
— Avg Daily Fat

WEEK

— BMI
— Miles Run

WEEK

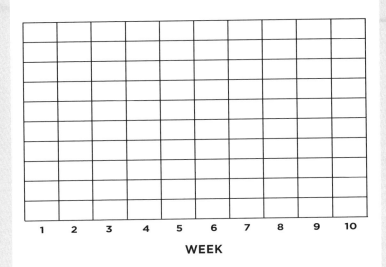

WEEK

1 2 3 4 5 6 7 8 9 10

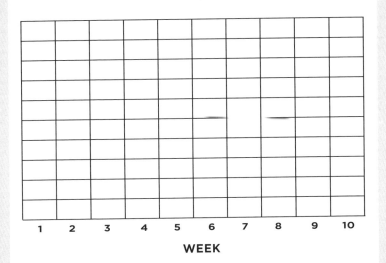

WEEK

1 2 3 4 5 6 7 8 9 10

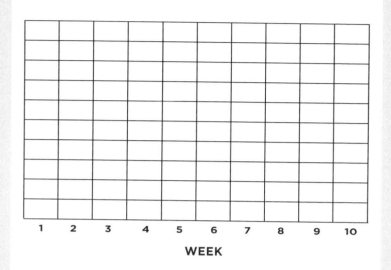

WEEK

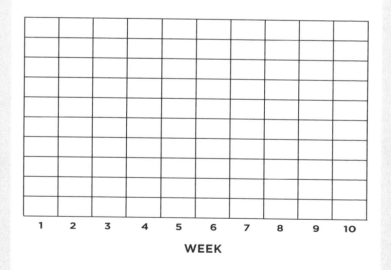

WEEK

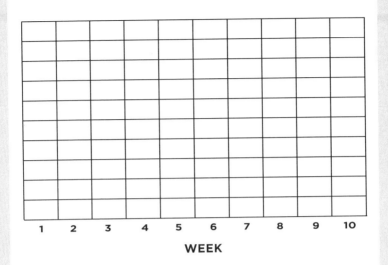

WEEK

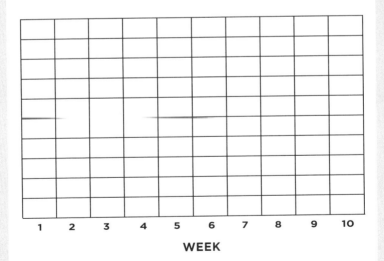

WEEK

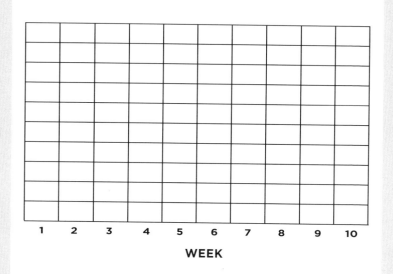

WEEK

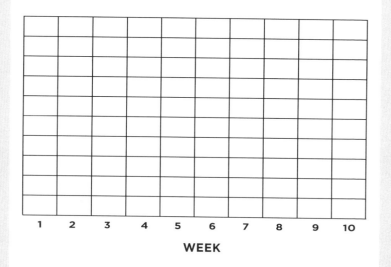

WEEK

Food & Fitness
REFERENCE
CHARTS

Exercise Chart

Estimated Calories Burned Per Hour Based On Body Weight[2]

ACTIVITY	130 LBS.	155 LBS.	190 LBS.
Aerobics, general	354	422	518
Aerobics, high impact	413	493	604
Aerobics, low impact	295	352	431
Archery (non-hunting)	207	246	302
Automobile repair	177	211	259
Backpacking, general	413	493	604
Basketball, game	472	563	690
Basketball, non-game, general	354	422	518
Basketball, wheelchair	384	457	561
Bicycling, < 10 mph, leisure	236	281	345
Bicycling, > 20 mph, racing	944	1,126	1,380
Bicycling, 10-11.9 mph, light effort	354	422	518
Bicycling, 12-13.9 mph, moderate effort	472	563	690
Bicycling, 14-15.9 mph, vigorous effort	590	704	863
Bicycling, 16-19 mph, very fast, racing	708	844	1035
Bicycling, BMX or mountain	502	598	733
Bicycling, stationary, light effort	325	387	474
Bicycling, stationary, moderate effort	413	493	604
Bicycling, stationary, vigorous effort	620	739	906
Billiards	148	176	216
Bowling	177	211	259

2   Department of Health and Family Services
Division of Public Health
PPH 40109 (09/05)
dhs.wisconsin.gov/publications/P4/p40109.pdf

ACTIVITY	130 LBS.	155 LBS.	190 LBS.
Boxing, in ring, general	708	844	1,035
Boxing, punching bag	354	422	518
Boxing, sparring	531	633	776
Calisthenics (push-ups, sit-ups), vigorous effort	472	563	690
Calisthenics, home, light/moderate effort	266	317	388
Canoeing, rowing, > 6 mph, vigorous effort	708	844	1,035
Canoeing, rowing, light effort	177	211	259
Canoeing, rowing, moderate effort	413	493	604
Carpentry, general	207	246	302
Child care: sitting, kneeling, dressing, feeding	177	211	259
Child care: standing-dressing, feeding	207	246	302
Cleaning, heavy, vigorous effort	266	317	388
Cleaning, house, general	207	246	302
Cleaning, light, moderate effort	148	176	216
Coaching: football, soccer, basketball, etc.	236	281	345
Cooking or food preparation	148	176	216
Dancing, aerobic, ballet or modern, twist	354	422	518
Dancing, ballroom, fast	325	387	474
Dancing, ballroom, slow	177	211	259
Dancing, general	266	317	388
Darts, wall or lawn	148	176	216
Diving, springboard or platform	177	211	259
Electrical work, plumbing	207	246	302
Farming, baling hay, cleaning barn	472	563	690

ACTIVITY	130 LBS.	155 LBS.	190 LBS.
Farming, shoveling grain	325	387	474
Fencing	354	422	518
Fishing from boat, sitting	148	176	216
Fishing from river bank, standing	207	246	302
Fishing in stream, in waders	354	422	518
Football or baseball, playing catch	148	176	216
Football, competitive	531	633	776
Football, touch, flag, general	472	563	690
Frisbee playing, general	177	211	259
Frisbee, ultimate	207	246	302
Gardening, general	295	352	431
Golf, carrying clubs	325	387	474
Golf, miniature or driving range	177	211	259
Golf, pulling clubs	295	352	431
Golf, using power cart	207	246	302
Gymnastics, general	236	281	345
Hacky sack	236	281	345
Hiking, cross country	354	422	518
Hockey, field	472	563	690
Hockey, ice	472	563	690
Horse grooming	354	422	518
Horse racing, galloping	472	563	690
Horseback riding, general	236	281	345
Horseback riding, trotting	384	457	561

ACTIVITY	130 LBS.	155 LBS.	190 LBS.
Horseback riding, walking	148	176	216
Hunting, general	295	352	431
Jogging, general	413	493	604
Judo, karate, kick boxing, tae kwan do	590	704	863
Kayaking	295	352	431
Kickball	413	493	604
Lacrosse	472	563	690
Marching band, playing instrument (walking)	236	281	345
Marching, rapidly, military	384	457	561
Motocross	236	281	345
Moving furniture, household	354	422	518
Moving household items, carrying boxes	413	493	604
Mowing lawn, general	325	387	474
Mowing lawn, riding mower	148	176	216
Music playing, cello, flute, horn, woodwind	118	141	173
Music playing, drums	236	281	345
Music playing, guitar, classical, folk (sitting)	118	141	173
Music playing, guitar, rock/roll band (standing)	177	211	259
Music playing, piano, organ, violin, trumpet	148	176	216
Painting, papering, plastering, scraping	266	317	388
Polo	472	563	690
Pushing or pulling stroller with child	148	176	216
Racquetball, casual, general	413	493	604
Racquetball, competitive	590	704	863

ACTIVITY	130 LBS.	155 LBS.	190 LBS.
Raking lawn	236	281	345
Rock climbing, ascending rock	649	774	949
Rock climbing, rappelling	472	563	690
Rope jumping, fast	708	844	1,035
Rope jumping, moderate, general	590	704	863
Rope jumping, slow	472	563	690
Rowing, stationary, light effort	561	669	819
Rowing, stationary, moderate effort	413	493	604
Rowing, stationary, vigorous effort	502	598	733
Rugby	590	704	863
Running, 10 mph (6-min. mile)	944	1,126	1,380
Running, 9 mph (6.5-min. mile)	885	1,056	1,294
Running, 8 mph (7.5-min. mile)	797	950	1,165
Running, 7 mph (8.5-min. mile)	679	809	992
Running, 6 mph (10-min. mile)	590	704	863
Running, 5 mph (12-min. mile)	472	563	690
Running, cross country	531	633	776
Running, general	472	563	690
Running, stairs, up	885	1,056	1,294
Sailing, boat/board, windsurfing, general	177	211	259
Sailing, in competition	295	352	431
Scrubbing floors, on hands and knees	325	387	474
Shoveling snow, by hand	354	422	518
Sitting-playing with children, light effort	148	176	216

ACTIVITY	130 LBS.	155 LBS.	190 LBS.
Skateboarding	295	352	431
Skating, ice, 9 mph or less	325	387	474
Skating, ice, general	413	493	604
Skating, ice, rapidly, > 9 mph	531	633	776
Skating, ice, speed, competitive	885	1,056	1,294
Skating, roller	413	493	604
Ski jumping (climb up carrying skis)	413	493	604
Ski machine, general	561	669	819
Skiing, cross-country, > 8.0 mph, racing	826	985	1,208
Skiing, cross-country, moderate effort	472	563	690
Skiing, cross-country, slow or light effort	413	493	604
Skiing, cross-country, vigorous effort	531	633	776
Skiing, downhill, light effort	295	352	431
Skiing, downhill, moderate effort	354	422	518
Skiing, downhill, vigorous effort, racing	472	563	690
Skiing, water	354	422	518
Ski-mobiling, water	413	493	604
Skin diving, scuba diving, general	413	493	604
Sledding, tobogganing, bobsledding, luge	413	493	604
Snorkeling	295	352	431
Snowshoeing	472	563	690
Snowmobiling	207	246	302
Soccer, casual, general	413	493	604
Soccer, competitive	590	704	863

ACTIVITY	130 LBS.	155 LBS.	190 LBS.
Softball or baseball, fast or slow pitch	295	352	431
Squash	708	844	1,035
Stair-treadmill ergometer, general	354	422	518
Stretching, hatha yoga	236	281	345
Surfing, body or board	177	211	259
Sweeping garage, sidewalk	236	281	345
Swimming laps, freestyle, fast, vigorous effort	590	704	863
Swimming laps, freestyle, light/moderate effort	472	563	690
Swimming, backstroke, general	472	563	690
Swimming, breaststroke, general	590	704	863
Swimming, butterfly, general	649	774	949
Swimming, leisurely, general	354	422	518
Swimming, sidestroke, general	472	563	690
Swimming, synchronized	472	563	690
Swimming, treading water, fast/vigorous	590	704	863
Swimming, treading water, moderate effort	236	281	345
Table tennis, ping pong	236	281	345
Tai chi	236	281	345
Tennis, doubles	354	422	518
Tennis, singles	472	563	690
Volleyball, beach	472	563	690
Volleyball, competitive, in gymnasium	236	281	345
Volleyball, noncompetitive; 6 to 9 member team	177	211	259
Walk/run-playing with children-moderate	236	281	345

ACTIVITY	130 LBS.	155 LBS.	190 LBS.
Walk/run-playing with children-vigorous	295	352	431
Walking, 2 mph, slow pace	148	176	216
Walking, 3 mph, moderate pace, walking dog	207	246	302
Walking, 3.5 mph, uphill	354	422	518
Walking, 4 mph, very brisk pace	236	281	345
Walking, carrying infant or 15-lb. load	207	246	302
Walking, grass track	295	352	431
Walking, upstairs	472	563	690
Water aerobics, water calisthenics	236	281	345
Water polo	590	704	863
Weight lifting or body building, vigorous effort	354	422	518
Weight lifting, light or moderate effort	177	211	259
Whitewater rafting, kayaking, or canoeing	295	352	431

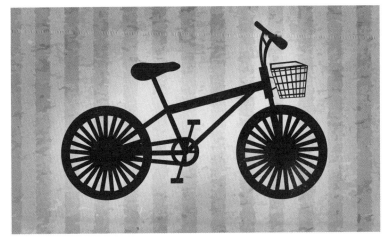

Fat & Calorie Chart
Nutritional Value Of Foods[2]

FOOD	AMOUNT	CALORIES	FAT (G)	SATURATED FAT (G)
BEVERAGES				
ALCOHOLIC				
BEER				
Regular	12 fl. oz.	146	0	0
Light	12 fl. oz.	99	0	0
GIN, RUM, VODKA, WHISKEY				
80 proof	1.5 fl. oz.	97	0	0
90 proof	1.5 fl. oz.	110	0	0
MIXED DRINKS				
Daiquiri	2 fl. oz.	112	trace	trace
Pina colada	4.5 fl. oz.	262	3	1.2
WINE				
Dessert				
Dry	3.5 fl. oz.	130	0	0
Sweet	3.5 fl. oz.	158	0	0
Table				
Red	3.5 fl. oz.	74	0	0
White	3.5 fl. oz.	70	0	0
CARBONATED				
CLUB SODA	12 fl. oz.	0	0	0
COLA TYPE	12 fl. oz.	152	0	0
DIET COLA (sweetened with aspartame)	12 fl. oz.	4	0	0
GINGER ALE	12 fl. oz.	124	0	0
LEMON LIME	12 fl. oz.	147	0	0
ORANGE	12 fl. oz.	179	0	0
ROOT BEER	12 fl. oz.	152	0	0
CHOCOLATE-FLAVORED BEVERAGE MIX				
POWDER	2-3 tsp.	75	1	0.4

3. Information taken from "Dietary Guidelines for Americans 2010"
   U.S. Department of Health and Human Services
   U.S. Department of Agriculture
   health.gov/dietaryguidelines/dga2010/DietaryGuidelines2010.pdf

FOOD	AMOUNT	CALORIES	FAT (G)	SATURATED FAT (G)
PREPARED WITH MILK	1 cup	226	9	5.5
COFFEE				
BREWED	6 fl. oz.	4	0	trace
ESPRESSO	2 fl. oz.	5	trace	0.1
INSTANT, PREPARED	6 fl. oz.	4	0	trace
MILK AND MILK BEVERAGES: *See Dairy Products*				
SOYMILK: *See Legumes, Nuts, and Seeds*				
TEA				
BREWED				
Black	6 fl. oz.	2	0	trace
Chamomile	6 fl. oz.	2	0	trace

DAIRY PRODUCTS

BUTTER: *See Fats and Oils*				
CHEESE / NATURAL				
BLUE	1 oz.	10	8	5.3
CAMEMBERT	1.32 oz.	114	9	5.8
CHEDDAR				
Cut pieces	1 oz.	114	8	6
Shredded	1 cup	455	37	23.8
COTTAGE				
Creamed (4% fat)				
Large-curd	1 cup	233	10	6.4
Small-curd	1 cup	217	9	6.0
Low-fat (2%)	1 cup	203	4	2.8
Low-fat (1%)	1 cup	164	2	1.5
Uncreamed (dry curd, less than ½% fat)	1 cup	123	1	0.4
CREAM				
Regular	1 oz.	99	10	6.2
	1 tbsp.	51	5	3.2
Low-fat	1 tbsp.	35	3	1.7

FOOD	AMOUNT	CALORIES	FAT (G)	SATURATED FAT (G)
Fat-free	1 tbsp.	15	trace	0.1
FETA	1 oz.	75	6	4.2
LOW-FAT, CHEDDAR OR COLBY	1 oz.	49	2	1.2
MOZZARELLA				
Whole milk	1 oz.	80	6	3.7
Part-skim milk (low moisture)	1 oz.	79	5	3.1
MUENSTER	1 oz.	104	9	5.4
PARMESAN, GRATED	1 cup	456	30	19.1
	1 tbsp.	23	2	1
	1 oz.	129	9	5.4
PROVOLONE	1 oz.	10	8	4.8
RICOTTA, MADE WITH				
Whole milk	1 cup	428	32	20.4
Part-skim milk	1 cup	340	19	12.1
SWISS	1 oz.	107	8	5
CREAM, SWEET				
HALF AND HALF	1 cup	315	28	17.3
	1 tbsp.	20	2	1.1
LIGHT, COFFEE, OR TABLE	1 cup	469	46	28.8
	1 tbsp.	29	3	1.8
WHIPPED TOPPING (pressurized)	1 cup	154	13	8.3
	1 tbsp.	8	1	0.4
CREAM, SOUR				
REGULAR	1 cup	493	48	3
	1 tbsp.	26	3	1.6
REDUCED-FAT	1 tbsp.	20	2	1.1
FAT-FREE	1 tbsp.	12	0	0
FROZEN DESSERT				
FROZEN YOGURT, SOFT-SERVE				
Chocolate	½ cup	115	4	2.6
Vanilla	½ cup	114	4	2.5

FOOD	AMOUNT	CALORIES	FAT (G)	SATURATED FAT (G)
ICE CREAM				
Regular				
Chocolate	½ cup	143	7	4.5
Vanilla	½ cup	133	7	4.5
50% reduced-fat vanilla	½ cup	92	3	1.7
Low-fat, chocolate	½ cup	113	2	1
Sherbet, orange	½ cup	102	1	0.9
MILK				
WHOLE (33% fat)	1 cup	150	8	5.1
REDUCED-FAT (2%)	1 cup	121	5	2.9
LOW-FAT (1%)	1 cup	102	3	1.6
NON-FAT (skim)	1 cup	86	trace	0.3
BUTTERMILK	1 cup	99	2	1.3
CANNED				
Condensed, sweetened	1 cup	982	27	16.8
Evaporated				
Whole milk	1 cup	339	19	11.6
Skim milk	1 cup	199	1	0.3
EGG				
RAW				
Whole	1 medium	66	4	1.4
	1 large	75	5	1.6
	1 extra large	86	6	1.8
White	1 large	17	0	0
Yoke	1 large	59	5	1.6
COOKED, WHOLE				
Fried, in margarine, with salt	1 large	92	7	1.9
Hard cooked, shell removed	1 large	78	6	1.6
Poached, with salt	1 large	75	5	1.5
Scrambled, in margarine, with whole milk, salt	1 large	101	7	2.2
EGG SUBSTITUTE	¼ cup	53	2	0.4

FOOD

	AMOUNT	CALORIES	FAT (G)	SATURATED FAT (G)
FATS AND OILS				
BUTTER (4 STICKS/LB.)				
SALTED	1 stick	813	92	57.3
	1 tbsp.	102	12	7.2
	1 tsp.	36	4	2.5
UNSALTED	1 stick	813	92	57.3
	1 tbsp.	115	13	5
MARGARINE				
REGULAR (about 80% fat)				
Hard (4 sticks/lb.)	1 stick	815	91	17.9
	1 tbsp.	101	11	2.2
	1 tsp.	34	4	0.7
Soft	1 cup	1,626	183	31.3
	1 tsp.	34	4	0.6
SPREAD (about 40% fat)	1 cup	801	90	17.9
	1 tsp.	17	2	0.4
OILS, SALAD OR COOKING				
CANOLA	1 tbsp.	124	14	1
OLIVE	1 tbsp.	119	14	1.8
PEANUT	1 tbsp.	119	14	2.3
SESAME	1 tbsp.	120	14	1.9
SOYBEAN, HYDROGENATED	1 tbsp.	120	14	2
SUNFLOWER	1 tbsp.	120	14	1.4
SALAD DRESSINGS / COMMERCIAL				
BLUE CHEESE				
Regular	1 tbsp.	77	8	1.5
Low-calorie	1 tbsp.	15	1	0.4
CAESAR				
Regular	1 tbsp.	78	8	1.3
Low-calorie	1 tbsp.	17	1	0.1

FOOD	AMOUNT	CALORIES	FAT (G)	SATURATED FAT (G)
FRENCH				
Regular	1 tbsp.	67	6	1.5
Low-calorie	1 tbsp.	22	1	0.1
ITALIAN				
Regular	1 tbsp.	69	7	1.0
Low-calorie	1 tbsp.	16	1	0.2
RUSSIAN				
Regular	1 tbsp.	76	8	1.1
Low-calorie	1 tbsp.	23	1	0.1
THOUSAND ISLAND				
Regular	1 tbsp.	59	6	0.9
Low-calorie	1 tbsp.	24	2	0.2
VINEGAR AND OIL	1 tbsp.	70	8	1.4

FISH AND SHELLFISH

FOOD	AMOUNT	CALORIES	FAT (G)	SATURATED FAT (G)
CATFISH, BREADED, FRIED	3 oz.	195	11	2.8
CLAM				
Raw, meat only	3 oz.	63	1	0.1
	1 medium	11	trace	trace
Breaded, fried	¾ cup	451	26	6.6
Canned, drained solids	3 oz.	126	2	0.2
	1 cup	237	3	0.3
COD				
Baked or broiled	3 oz.	89	1	0.1
CRAB				
Alaska King				
Steamed	1 leg	130	2	0.2
	3 oz.	82	1	0.1
Imitation	3 oz.	87	1	0.2
Blue				
Steamed	3 oz.	87	2	0.2
Canned	1 cup	134	2	0.3

FOOD	AMOUNT	CALORIES	FAT (G)	SATURATED FAT (G)
CRAB CAKE (with egg, onion, fried in margarine)	1 cake	93	5	0.9
FISH FILLET (battered or breaded, fried)	1 fillet	211	11	2.6
FISH STICK (breaded)	1 stick	76	3	0.9
FLOUNDER OR SOLE (baked or broiled)	3 oz.	99	1	0.3
	1 fillet	149	2	0.5
HADDOCK (baked or broiled)	3 oz.	95	1	0.1
	1 fillet	168	1	0.3
HALIBUT (baked or broiled)	3 oz.	119	2	0.4
	½ fillet	223	5	0.7
HERRING (pickled)	3 oz.	223	15	2
LOBSTER (steamed)	3 oz.	83	1	0.1
OYSTER				
Raw, meat only	1 cup	169	6	1.9
	6 medium	57	2	0.6
Breaded, fried	3 oz.	167	11	2.7
POLLOCK (baked or broiled)	3 oz.	96	1	0.2
	1 fillet	68	1	0.1
ROCKFISH (baked or broiled)	3 oz.	103	2	0.4
	1 fillet	180	3	0.7
SALMON				
Baked or broiled	3 oz.	184	9	1.6
	½ fillet	335	17	3.0
Canned (pink)	3 oz.	118	5	1.3
Smoked (Chinook)	3 oz.	99	4	0.8
SARDINE, ATLANTIC (canned in oil, drained solids)	3 oz.	177	10	1.3
SCALLOP				
Breaded, fried	6 large	20	10	2.5
Steamed	3 oz.	95	1	0.1
SHRIMP				
Breaded, fried	3 oz.	206	10	1.8
	6 large	109	6	0.9

FOOD	AMOUNT	CALORIES	FAT (G)	SATURATED FAT (G)
Canned	3 oz.	102	2	0.3
TROUT (baked or broiled)	3 oz.	144	6	1.8
	1 fillet	120	5	1.5
TUNA				
Baked or broiled	3 oz.	118	1	0.3
Canned				
Oil-pack, light	3 oz.	168	7	1.3
Water-pack, light	3 oz.	99	1	0.2
Water-pack, solid	3 oz.	109	3	0.7

FRUITS AND FRUIT JUICES

APPLES				
Raw				
Unpeeled	1 apple	81	trace	0.1
Peeled, sliced	1 cup	63	trace	0.1
Dried	5 rings	78	trace	trace
Apple juice	1 cup	117	trace	trace
Applesauce, canned				
Sweetened	1 cup	194	trace	0.1
Unsweetened	1 cup	105	trace	trace
APRICOTS				
Raw	1 apricot	17	trace	trace
Canned				
Heavy syrup pack	1 cup	214	trace	trace
Dried, sulfured	10 halves	83	trace	trace
ASIAN PEAR, RAW (3⅜" high x 3")	1 pear	116	1	trace
AVOCADOS (raw, without skin and seed)				
California (about ⅕ whole)	1 oz.	50	5	0.7
Florida (about ⅒ whole)	1 oz.	32	3	0.5
BANANAS, RAW				
Whole, medium	1 banana	109	1	0.2

FOOD	AMOUNT	CALORIES	FAT (G)	SATURATED FAT (G)
BLACKBERRIES, RAW	1 cup	75	1	trace
BLUEBERRIES				
Raw	1 cup	81	1	trace
Frozen, sweetened, thawed	1 cup	186	trace	trace
CANTALOUPE (5" diameter)				
Wedge	⅛ melon	24	trace	trace
Cubes	1 cup	56	trace	0.1
CHERRIES				
Sour, red, pitted, canned, water-pack	1 cup	88	trace	0.1
Sweet, raw, without pits and stems	10 cherries	49	1	0.1
CRANBERRIES				
Dried, sweetened	¼ cup	92	trace	trace
CRANBERRY SAUCE, canned (about 8 slices per can)	1 slice	86	trace	trace
CRANBERRY JUICE	8 fl. oz.	144	trace	trace
DATES (without pits)				
Whole	5 dates	116	trace	0.1
Chopped	1 cup	490	1	0.3
FIGS, dried	2 figs	97	trace	0.1
FRUIT COCKTAIL (canned, fruit and liquid)				
Heavy syrup pack	1 cup	181	trace	trace
Juice pack	1 cup	109	trace	trace
GRAPEFRUIT				
Pink or red	½ grapefruit	37	trace	trace
Canned, sections with light syrup	1 cup	152	trace	trace
GRAPEFRUIT JUICE				
Raw	1 cup	96	trace	trace
Canned				
Unsweetened	1 cup	94	trace	trace
Sweetened	1 cup	115	trace	trace
GRAPES, RAW	10 grapes	36	trace	0.1
	1 cup	114	1	0.3

FOOD	AMOUNT	CALORIES	FAT (G)	SATURATED FAT (G)
HONEYDEW (6"-7" diameter)				
Wedge	⅛ melon	56	trace	trace
Diced	1 cup	60	trace	trace
KIWI FRUIT, RAW (without skin)	1 medium	46	trace	trace
LEMONS, RAW (peeled)	1 lemon	17	trace	trace
LEMON JUICE				
Raw	1 lemon	12	0	0
Canned or bottled	1 tbsp.	3	trace	trace
LIME JUICE				
Raw	1 lime	10	trace	trace
Canned	1 tbsp.	3	trace	trace
MANGOES, RAW (skinned, and seeded)				
Whole	1 mango	135	1	0.1
Sliced	1 cup	107	trace	0.1
NECTARINES, RAW (2½" diameter)	1 nectarine	67	1	0.1
ORANGES				
Whole	1 orange	62	trace	trace
Sections	1 cup	85	trace	trace
ORANGE JUICE	1 cup	112	trace	0.1
PEACHES				
Raw				
Whole	1 peach	42	trace	trace
Sliced	1 cup	73	trace	trace
Canned				
Heavy syrup	1 cup	194	trace	trace
Dried, sulfured	3 halves	93	trace	trace
PEARS				
Raw	1 pear	98	1	trace
Canned, fruit and liquid				
Heavy syrup pack	1 cup	197	trace	trace

FOOD	AMOUNT	CALORIES	FAT (G)	SATURATED FAT (G)
PINEAPPLE				
Raw, diced	1 cup	76	1	trace
Canned, fruit and liquid				
Slices (3" diameter)	1 slice	38	trace	trace
PINEAPPLE JUICE (unsweetened)	1 cup	140	trace	trace
PLANTAIN, PEELED				
Raw	1 medium	218	1	0.3
Cooked, slices	1 cup	179	trace	0.1
PLUMS, RAW (2-⅛" diameter)	1 plum	36	trace	trace
PRUNES, DRIED, PITTED				
Uncooked	5 prunes	10	trace	trace
Stewed	1 cup	265	1	trace
PRUNE JUICE (canned or bottled)	1 cup	182	trace	trace
RAISINS (seedless)	1 cup	435	1	0.2
RASPBERRIES				
Raw	1 cup	60	1	trace
Frozen	1 cup	258	trace	trace
RHUBARB (cooked with sugar)	1 cup	278	trace	trace
STRAWBERRIES				
Large	1 strawberry	5	trace	trace
Medium	1 strawberry	4	trace	trace
Sliced	1 cup	50	1	trace
Frozen	1 cup	245	trace	trace
TANGERINES, RAW	1 tangerine	37	trace	trace
Canned (mandarin), light syrup, fruit and liquid	1 cup	154	trace	trace
WATERMELON, DICED	1 cup	49	1	0.1

FOOD	AMOUNT	CALORIES	FAT (G)	SATURATED FAT (G)
GRAIN PRODUCTS				
BAGELS, ENRICHED				
PLAIN	4" bagel	245	1	0.2
CINNAMON RAISIN	4" bagel	244	2	0.2
EGG	4" bagel	247	2	0.4
BREADS				
BANANA BREAD	1 slice	196	6	1.3
BISCUITS (plain or buttermilk, enriched)	2½" biscuit	212	10	2.6
	4" biscuit	358	16	4.4
ENRICHED				
Cracked wheat	1 slice	65	1	0.2
Egg bread (challah)	½" slice	115	2	0.6
French or Vienna (also sourdough)	½" slice	69	1	0.2
Italian	1 slice	54	1	0.2
ENGLISH MUFFIN	1 muffin	134	1	0.1
MIXED GRAIN BREAD	1 slice	65	1	0.2
OAT	1 slice	73	1	0.2
PITA	4" pita	77	trace	trace
	6 ½" pita	165	1	0.1
PUMPERNICKEL	1 slice	80	1	0.1
RYE	1 slice	83	1	0.2
WHEAT	1 slice	65	1	0.2
WHITE	1 slice	67	1	0.1
WHOLE WHEAT	1 slice	69	1	0.3
BREAD CRUMBS				
DRY, GRATED				
Plain, enriched	1 cup	427	6	1.3
Seasoned, unenriched	1 cup	440	3	0.9
BREAD STUFFING (prepared from dry mix)	½ cup	178	9	1.7

FOOD	AMOUNT	CALORIES	FAT (G)	SATURATED FAT (G)
BROWNIES				
REGULAR (large)	1 brownie	227	9	2.4
FAT-FREE (2" sq.)	1 brownie	89	trace	0.2
REDUCED-CALORIE (2" sq.)	1 brownie	84	2	1.1
BULGUR				
UNCOOKED	1 cup	479	2	0.3
COOKED	1 cup	151	trace	0.1
CAKES				
CAKES, PREPARED FROM DRY MIX				
Angel food (1/12 of 10" cake)	1 piece	129	trace	trace
Yellow, light, egg whites, no frosting (1/12 of 9" cake)	1 piece	181	2	1.1
CAKES, PREPARED FROM RECIPE				
Chocolate, without frosting (1/12 of 9" diameter)	1 piece	340	14	5.2
Pineapple upside down (1/9 of 8" square)	1 piece	367	14	3.4
Sponge (1/12 of 16-oz. cake)	1 piece	187	3	0.8
White without frosting (1/12 of 9" diameter)	1 piece	264	9	2
CAKES, COMMERCIALLY PREPARED				
Angel food (1/12 of 12-oz. cake)	1 piece	72	trace	trace
Chocolate, chocolate frosting (1/8 of 18-oz. cake)	1 piece	235	10	3.1
Coffeecake, crumb (1/9 of 20-oz. cake)	1 piece	263	15	3.7
POUND				
Butter (1 1/12 of 12-oz. cake)	1 piece	109	6	3.2
Fat-free (3¼" x 2¾" x ⅝" slice)	1 slice	79	trace	0.1
SNACK CAKES				
Sponge	1 shortcake	87	1	0.2
Yellow				
With chocolate frosting	1 piece	243	11	3
With vanilla frosting	1 piece	239	9	1.5
CHEESECAKE (1/6 of 17-oz. cake)	1 piece	257	18	7.9
COOKIES				
BUTTER (commercially prepared)	1 cookie	23	1	0.6

FOOD	AMOUNT	CALORIES	FAT (G)	SATURATED FAT (G)
CHOCOLATE CHIP, MEDIUM (2¼"-2½" DIAMETER)				
Commercially prepared	1 cookie	48	2	0.7
From refrigerated dough	1 cookie	128	6	2
Prepared from recipe, with margarine	1 cookie	78	5	1.3
OATMEAL				
Commercially prepared, with or without raisins				
Regular, large	1 cookie	113	5	1.1
Soft-type	1 cookie	61	2	0.5
Fat-free	1 cookie	36	trace	trace
Prepared from recipe, with raisins (2⅝" diameter)	1 cookie	65	2	0.5
PEANUT BUTTER				
Commercially prepared	1 cookie	72	4	0.7
Prepared from recipe, with margarine (3" diameter)	1 cookie	95	5	0.9
SANDWICH-TYPE, WITH CREAM FILLING				
Chocolate	1 cookie	47	2	0.4
Vanilla cookie, oval	1 cookie	72	3	0.4
SHORTBREAD (commercially prepared)				
Plain (1⅝" square)	1 cookie	40	2	0.5
SUGAR				
Commercially prepared	1 cookie	72	3	0.8
From refrigerated dough	1 cookie	73	3	0.9
Prepared from recipe, margarine (3" diameter)	1 cookie	66	3	0.7
VANILLA WAFER, LOWER-FAT, MEDIUM SIZE	1 cookie	18	1	0.2
CORN CHIPS				
Plain	1 oz.	153	9	1.3
CORNBREAD				
Prepared from mix	1 piece	188	6	1.6
COUSCOUS				
Uncooked	1 cup	650	1	0.2
Cooked	1 cup	176	trace	trace

FOOD	AMOUNT	CALORIES	FAT (G)	SATURATED FAT (G)
CRACKERS				
CHEESE (1" diameter)	10 crackers	50	3	0.9
GRAHAM, PLAIN				
2½" square	2 squares	59	1	0.2
Crushed	1 cup	355	8	1.3
MELBA TOAST, PLAIN	4 pieces	78	1	0.1
SALTINE				
Square	4 crackers	52	1	0.4
Oyster-type	1 cup	195	5	1.3
STANDARD SNACK TYPE				
Round	4 crackers	60	3	0.5
Wheat, square	4 crackers	38	2	0.4
DANISH PASTRY, ENRICHED				
CHEESE-FILLED	1 Danish	266	16	4.8
FRUIT-FILLED	1 Danish	263	13	3.5
DOUGHNUTS				
CAKE-TYPE	1 hole	59	3	0.5
	1 medium	198	11	1.7
YEAST (leavened, glazed)	1 hole	52	3	0.8
	1 medium	242	14	3.5
ÉCLAIR	1 éclair	262	16	4.1
GRANOLA BAR				
HARD (plain)	1 bar	134	6	0.7
SOFT (uncoated chocolate chip)	1 bar	119	5	2.9
RAISIN	1 bar	127	5	2.7
MATZO				
PLAIN	1 matzo	112	trace	0.1
MUFFINS (2½" X 2½")				
BLUEBERRY				
Commercially prepared	1 muffin	158	4	0.8
Prepared from recipe	1 muffin	162	6	1.2

FOOD	AMOUNT	CALORIES	FAT (G)	SATURATED FAT (G)
CORN				
Commercially prepared	1 muffin	174	5	0.8
Prepared from mix	1 muffin	161	5	1.4
OAT BRAN (commercially prepared)	1 muffin	154	4	0.6
NOODLES				
EGG NOODLES (enriched, cooked)	1 cup	213	2	0.5
MACARONI (elbows, enriched, cooked)	1 cup	197	1	0.1
OAT BRAN				
Uncooked	1 cup	231	7	1.2
Cooked	1 cup	88	2	0.4
PANCAKES, PLAIN (4″ DIAMETER)				
Prepared from complete mix	1 pancake	74	1	0.2
Prepared from incomplete mix, (2% milk, egg, oil)	1 pancake	83	3	0.8
PIES				
PREPARED FROM RECIPE (⅛ OF 9″ diameter)				
Apple	1 piece	411	19	4.7
Blueberry	1 piece	360	17	4.3
Cherry	1 piece	486	22	5.4
Lemon meringue	1 piece	362	16	4
Pecan	1 piece	503	27	4.9
Pumpkin	1 piece	316	14	4.9
POPCORN				
AIR-POPPED (plain)	1 cup	31	trace	trace
OIL-POPPED (salted)	1 cup	55	3	0.5
CARAMEL-COATED				
with peanuts	1 cup	168	3	0.4
without peanuts	1 cup	152	5	1.3
CHEESE-FLAVORED	1 cup	58	4	0.7
PRETZELS, MADE WITH ENRICHED FLOUR				
STICK (2¼″ long)	10 pretzels	11	trace	trace
TWISTED, REGULAR	10 pretzels	229	2	0.5

FOOD	AMOUNT	CALORIES	FAT (G)	SATURATED FAT (G)
TWISTED, DUTCH (soft)	1 pretzel	61	1	0.1
RICE				
BROWN, LONG GRAIN, COOKED	1 cup	216	2	0.4
Raw	1 cup	675	1	0.3
Cooked	1 cup	205	trace	0.1
Instant, prepared	1 cup	162	trace	0.1
ROLL				
DINNER	1 roll	84	2	0.5
HAMBURGER/HOTDOG	1 roll	123	2	0.5
HARD, KAISER	1 roll	167	2	0.3
SPAGHETTI, COOKED				
ENRICHED	1 cup	197	1	0.1
WHOLE WHEAT	1 cup	174	1	0.1
SWEET ROLLS, CINNAMON				
COMMERCIAL (with raisins)	1 roll	223	10	1.8
REFRIGERATED DOUGH (baked, with frosting)	1 roll	109	4	1
TACO SHELL				
BAKED	1 medium	62	3	0.4
TORTILLA CHIPS				
PLAIN				
Regular	1 oz.	142	7	14
Low-fat, baked	10 chips	54	1	0.1
WAFFLES, PLAIN				
Prepared from recipe, 7" diameter	1 waffle	218	11	2.1
Frozen, toasted, 4" diameter	1 waffle	87	3	0.5
WHEAT FLOURS				
ALL-PURPOSE, ENRICHED				
Sifted, spooned	1 cup	419	1	0.2
Unsifted, spooned	1 cup	455	1	0.2
BREAD, ENRICHED	1 cup	495	2	0.3
CAKE OR PASTRY FLOUR (enriched, unsifted, spooned)	1 cup	496	1	0.2

FOOD	AMOUNT	CALORIES	FAT (G)	SATURATED FAT (G)
SELF-RISING (enriched, unsifted, spooned)	1 cup	443	1	0.2
WHOLE WHEAT (from hard wheat, stirred, spooned)	1 cup	407	2	0.4

LEGUMES, NUTS, AND SEEDS

ALMONDS, SHELLED

Sliced	1 cup	549	48	3.7
Whole	1 oz. (24 nuts)	164	14	1.1

BEANS, DRY

Cooked				
Black	1 cup	227	1	0.2
Great Northern	1 cup	209	1	0.2
Kidney, red	1 cup	225	1	0.1
Lima, large	1 cup	216	1	0.2
Pea (navy)	1 cup	258	1	0.3
Pinto	1 cup	234	1	0.2
Canned, solids and liquid				
Baked beans				
Plain or vegetarian	1 cup	236	1	0.3
With pork in tomato sauce	1 cup	248	3	1
With pork in sweet sauce	1 cup	281	4	1.4
Kidney, red	1 cup	218	1	0.1
Lima, large	1 cup	190	trace	0.1
White	1 cup	307	1	0.2

BLACK-EYED PEAS

Cooked	1 cup	20	1	0.2
Canned, solids and liquid	1 cup	185	1	0.3
BRAZIL NUTS, SHELLED	1 oz. (6-8 nuts)	186	19	4.6

CASHEWS, SALTED

Dry-roasted	1 oz.	163	13	2.6
Oil-roasted	1 cup	749	63	12.4
CHESTNUTS, EUROPEAN (roasted, shelled)	1 cup	350	3	0.6

FOOD	AMOUNT	CALORIES	FAT (G)	SATURATED FAT (G)
CHICKPEAS				
Cooked	1 cup	269	4	0.4
Canned, solids and liquid	1 cup	286	3	0.3
COCONUT				
Raw				
Piece, about 2" x 2" x ½"	1 piece	159	15	13.4
Shredded, not packed	1 cup	283	27	23.8
Dried, sweetened, shredded	1 cup	466	33	29.3
HAZELNUTS (filberts), chopped	1 cup	722	70	5.1
LENTILS dry, cooked	1 cup	230	1	0.1
MACADAMIA NUTS, dry-roasted, salted	1 cup	959	102	16
MIXED NUTS				
Dry-roasted	1 oz.	168	15	2
Oil-roasted	1 oz.	175	16	2.5
PEANUTS				
Dry-roasted				
Salted	1 oz. (about 28)	166	14	2
Unsalted	1 oz. (about 28)	166	14	2
Oil-roasted, salted	1 oz.	165	14	1.9
PEANUT BUTTER				
Regular				
Smooth-style	1 tbsp.	95	8	1.7
Chunky-style	1 tbsp.	94	8	1.5
Reduced-fat	1 tbsp.	94	6	1.3
PEAS, SPLIT (dry, cooked)	1 cup	231	1	0.1
PECANS, HALVES	1 cup	746	78	6.7
PINE NUTS, SHELLED	1 oz.	160	14	2.2
PISTACHIO NUTS (dry-roasted, with salt, shelled)	1 oz.	161	13	1.6
PUMPKIN AND SQUASH KERNELS (roasted, with salt)	1 oz.	148	12	2.3
REFRIED BEANS (canned)	1 cup	237	3	1.2

FOOD

FOOD	AMOUNT	CALORIES	FAT (G)	SATURATED FAT (G)
Sesame seeds	1 tbsp.	47	4	0.6
Soybeans (dry, cooked)	1 cup	298	15	2.2
Sunflower seed kernels (dry-roasted, with salt)	¼ cup	186	16	1.7
	1 oz.	165	14	1.5
Tahini	1 tbsp.	89	8	1.1
Walnuts, English	1 cup	785	78	7.4

MEAT AND MEAT PRODUCTS

BEEF, COOKED

Cuts braised, simmered, or pot-roasted

Relatively fat, such as chuck blade, piece, 2½" x 2½" x ¾"				
Lean and fat	3 oz.	293	22	8.7
Lean only	3 oz.	213	11	4.3
Relatively lean, such as bottom round, piece, 4⅛" x 2¼" x ½"				
Lean and fat	3 oz.	234	14	5.4
Lean only	3 oz.	178	7	2.4

Ground beef, broiled

83% lean	3 oz.	218	14	5.5
79% lean	3 oz.	231	16	6.2
73% lean	3 oz.	246	18	6.9

Roast, oven cooked, no liquid added

Relatively fat, such as rib, 2 pieces, 4⅛" x 2¼" x ¼"				
Lean and fat	3 oz.	304	25	9.9
Lean only	3 oz.	195	11	4.2
Relatively lean, such as eye of round, 2 pieces, 2½" x 2½" x ⅜"				
Lean and fat	3 oz.	195	11	4.2
Lean only	3 oz.	143	4	1.5

Steak, sirloin, broiled, piece, 2½" x 2½" x ¾"

Lean and fat	3 oz.	219	13	5.2
Lean only	3 oz.	166	6	2.4

FOOD

	AMOUNT	CALORIES	FAT (G)	SATURATED FAT (G)
LAMB, COOKED				
CHOPS				
Loin, broiled				
Lean and fat	3 oz.	269	20	8.4
Lean only	3 oz.	184	8	3
Leg, roasted, 2 pieces, 4⅛" x 2¼" x ¼"				
Lean and fat	3 oz.	219	14	5.9
Lean only	3 oz.	162	7	2.3
Rib, roasted, 3 pieces, 2½" x 2½" x ¼"				
Lean and fat	3 oz.	305	25	10.9
Lean only	3 oz.	197	11	4
PORK, CURED, COOKED				
BACON				
Regular	3 slices	109	9	3.3
Canadian style (6 slices per 6-oz. pack.)	2 slices	86	4	1.3
HAM, LIGHT CURE, ROASTED, 2 PIECES, 4⅛" x 2¼" x ¼"				
Lean and fat	3 oz.	207	14	5.1
Lean only	3 oz.	133	5	1.6
PORK, FRESH, COOKED				
Broiled				
Lean and fat	3 oz.	204	11	4.1
Lean only	3 oz.	172	7	2.5
Pan-fried				
Lean and fat	3 oz.	235	14	5.1
Lean only	3 oz.	197	9	3.1
HAM (LEG), ROASTED, PIECE, 2½" x 2½" x ¾"				
Lean and fat	3 oz.	232	15	5.5
Lean only	3 oz.	179	8	2.8
RIB ROAST, PIECE, 2½" x 2½" x ¾"				
Lean and fat	3 oz.	217	13	5

FOOD	AMOUNT	CALORIES	FAT (G)	SATURATED FAT (G)
Lean only	3 oz.	190	9	3.7
RIBS, LEAN AND FAT, COOKED				
Backribs, roasted	3 oz.	315	25	9.3
Country-style, braised	3 oz.	252	18	6.8
Spareribs, braised	3 oz.	337	26	9.5
SHOULDER CUT, BRAISED, 3 pieces, 2½" x 2½" x ¼"				
Lean and fat	3 oz.	280	20	7.2
Lean only	3 oz.	211	10	3.5
SAUSAGES				
BOLOGNA, BEEF AND PORK (8 slices per 8-oz. pack)	2 slices	180	16	6.1
BROWN AND SERVE, COOKED, LINK, 4" x ⅞" raw	2 links	103	9	3.4
FRANKFURTER (10 per 1-lb. pack, heated)				
Beef and pork	1 frank	144	13	4.8
Beef	1 frank	142	13	5.4
PORK SAUSAGE, FRESH, COOKED				
Link	2 links	96	8	2.8
Patty	1 patty	10	8	2.9
SALAMI, BEEF AND PORK				
Cooked type (8 slices per 8-oz. pack)	2 slices	143	11	4.6
Dry type, sliced, 3⅛" x ¹⁄₁₆"	2 slices	84	7	2.4
VIENNA SAUSAGE (7 per 4-oz. can)	1 sausage	45	4	1.5
FAST FOODS				
BREAKFAST ITEMS				
Biscuit with egg, sausage	1 biscuit	581	39	15
Croissant with egg, cheese, bacon	1 croissant	413	28	15.4
Danish pastry				
Cheese-filled	1 pastry	353	25	5.1
Fruit-filled	1 pastry	335	16	3.3
ENGLISH MUFFIN (egg, cheese, Canadian bacon)	1 muffin	289	13	4.7
HASHED BROWN POTATOES	½ cup	151	9	4.3

FOOD	AMOUNT	CALORIES	FAT (G)	SATURATED FAT (G)
BURRITO				
Beans and cheese	1 burrito	189	6	3.4
Beans and meat	1 burrito	255	9	4.2
CHEESEBURGER				
Regular size, with condiments				
Double patty with mayo, vegetables	1 sandwich	417	21	8.7
Single patty	1 sandwich	295	14	6.3
Single patty with bacon	1 sandwich	608	37	16.2
CHICKEN FILLET (breaded and fried, plain)	1 sandwich	515	29	8.5
CHICKEN PIECES, BONELESS (breaded and fried, plain)	6 pieces	319	21	4.7
ENCHILADA WITH CHEESE	1 enchilada	319	19	10.6
FISH SANDWICH (with tartar sauce and cheese)	1 sandwich	523	29	8.1
FRENCH FRIES	1 small	291	16	3.3
	1 medium	458	25	5.2
	1 large	578	31	6.5
HAMBURGER				
Regular size, with condiments				
Double patty	1 sandwich	576	32	12
Single patty	1 sandwich	272	10	3.6
HOT DOG				
CORNDOG	1 corndog	460	19	5.2
Plain	1 corndog	242	15	5.1
With chili	1 corndog	296	13	4.9
ONION RINGS (breaded and fried)	8-9 rings	276	16	7
PIZZA (slice = ⅛ of 12" pizza)				
Cheese	1 slice	140	3	1.5
Meat and vegetables	1 slice	184	5	1.5
Pepperoni	1 slice	181	7	2.2
SHAKE				
Chocolate	16 fl. oz.	423	12	7.7
Vanilla	16 fl. oz.	370	10	6.2

FOOD	AMOUNT	CALORIES	FAT (G)	SATURATED FAT (G)
SHRIMP (breaded and fried)	6-8 shrimp	454	25	5.4
SUBMARINE SANDWICH (6", with oil and vinegar)				
Cold cuts (lettuce, cheese, salami, ham, tomato)	1 sandwich	456	19	6.8
Roast beef (with tomato, lettuce, mayo)	1 sandwich	410	13	7.1
Tuna salad (with mayo, lettuce)	1 sandwich	584	28	5.3
TACO, BEEF	1 small	369	21	11.4

POULTRY AND POULTRY PRODUCTS

CHICKEN

FRIED IN VEGETABLE SHORTENING (meat with skin)

Batter-dipped				
Breast	½ breast	364	18	4.9
Drumstick	1 drumstick	193	11	3
Thigh	1 thigh	238	14	3.8
Wing	1 wing	159	11	2.9
FLOUR-COATED				
Breast	½ breast	218	9	2.4
Drumstick	1 drumstick	120	7	1.8
FRIED, MEAT ONLY				
Dark meat	3 oz.	203	10	2.7
Light meat	3 oz.	163	5	1.3
ROASTED, MEAT ONLY				
Breast	½ breast	142	3	0.9
Drumstick	1 drumstick	76	2	0.7
Thigh	1 thigh	109	6	1.6

DUCK

ROASTED, MEAT ONLY	½ duck	444	25	9.2

TURKEY

ROASTED, MEAT ONLY				
Dark meat	3 oz.	159	6	2.1
Light meat	3 oz.	133	3	0.9

FOOD

	AMOUNT	CALORIES	FAT (G)	SATURATED FAT (G)
SOUPS, SAUCES, AND GRAVIES				
SOUPS				
HOME-PREPARED STOCK				
Beef	1 cup	31	trace	0.1
Chicken	1 cup	86	3	0.8
Fish	1 cup	40	2	0.5
SAUCES				
READY-TO-SERVE				
Barbecue	1 tbsp.	12	trace	trace
Cheese	¼ cup	110	8	3.8
Pepper or hot	1 tsp.	90	trace	trace
Salsa	1 tbsp.	4	trace	trace
Soy	1 tbsp.	9	trace	trace
Spaghetti/marinara/pasta	1 cup	143	5	0.7
Teriyaki	1 tbsp.	15	0	0
Worcestershire	1 tbsp.	11	0	0
GRAVIES, CANNED				
Beef	¼ cup	31	1	0.7
Chicken	¼ cup	47	3	0.8
Country sausage	¼ cup	96	8	2
Mushroom	¼ cup	30	2	0.2
Turkey	¼ cup	31	1	0.4
SUGARS AND SWEETS				
CARAMEL				
Plain	1 piece	39	1	0.7
Chocolate-flavored	1 piece	25	trace	trace
CHOCOLATE CHIPS				
Milk	1 cup	862	52	31
Semisweet	1 cup	805	50	29.8
White	1 cup	916	55	33

FOOD	AMOUNT	CALORIES	FAT (G)	SATURATED FAT (G)
CHOCOLATE-COATED PEANUTS	10 pieces	208	13	5.8
CHOCOLATE-COATED RAISINS	10 pieces	39	1	0.9
FRUIT LEATHER, ROLLS	1 large	74	1	0.1
	1 small	49	trace	0.1
FUDGE, PREPARED FROM RECIPE				
Chocolate	1 piece	65	1	0.9
Vanilla	1 piece	59	1	0.5
GUMMY BEARS	10 bears	85	0	0
HARD CANDY	1 piece	24	trace	0
JELLY BEANS	10 large	104	trace	trace
MARSHMALLOWS				
Miniature	1 cup	159	trace	trace
Regular	1 regular	23	trace	trace
FROZEN DESSERTS (nondairy)				
Fruit and juice bar	1 bar (2.5 fl. oz.)	63	trace	0
Ice pop	1 bar (2 fl. oz.)	42	0	0
Italian ices	½ cup	86	trace	0
GELATIN DESSERT (prepared with powder and water)				
Regular	½ cup	80	0	0
Reduced calorie (with aspartame)	½ cup	8	0	0
HONEY, STRAINED OR EXTRACTED	1 tbsp.	64	0	0
JAMS AND PRESERVES	1 tbsp.	56	trace	trace
JELLIES	1 tbsp.	54	trace	trace
PUDDINGS				
Chocolate	½ cup	150	3	1.6
Vanilla	½ cup	148	2	1.4
SUGAR				
Brown				
Packed	1 cup	827	0	0
Unpacked	1 cup	545	0	0
White				

FOOD	AMOUNT	CALORIES	FAT (G)	SATURATED FAT (G)
Granulated	1 packet	23	0	0
	1 tsp.	16	0	0
Powdered, unsifted	1 tbsp.	31	trace	trace
SYRUP				
Chocolate-flavored syrup or topping				
Thin type	1 tbsp.	53	trace	0.1
Fudge type	1 tbsp.	67	2	0.8
Corn, light	1 tbsp.	56	0	0
Maple	1 tbsp.	52	trace	trace

VEGETABLES AND VEGETABLE PRODUCTS

FOOD	AMOUNT	CALORIES	FAT (G)	SATURATED FAT (G)
ALFALFA SPROUTS, RAW	1 cup	10	trace	trace
ARTICHOKES (globe or French, cooked, drained)	1 medium	60	trace	trace
ASPARAGUS, GREEN				
Cooked, drained				
From raw	1 cup	43	1	0.1
	4 spears	14	trace	trace
From frozen	1 cup	50	1	0.2
	4 spears	17	trace	0.1
Canned, spears about 5" long, drained	1 cup	46	2	0.4
	4 spears	14	trace	0.1
BEANS				
Lima, immature seeds, frozen, cooked, drained				
Fordhooks	1 cup	170	1	0.1
Baby limas	1 cup	189	1	0.1
Snap, cut				
Cooked, drained				
From raw	1 cup	44	trace	0.1
From frozen	1 cup	38	trace	0.1
Canned, drained	1 cup	27	trace	trace

FOOD	AMOUNT	CALORIES	FAT (G)	SATURATED FAT (G)
BEANS, DRY: SEE LEGUMES				
BEAN SPROUTS (mung)				
Raw	1 cup	31	trace	trace
Cooked, drained	1 cup	26	trace	trace
BEETS				
Cooked, drained				
Slices	1 cup	75	trace	trace
Whole beet, 2"	1 beet	22	trace	trace
Canned, drained				
Slices	1 cup	53	trace	trace
Whole beet	1 beet	7	trace	trace
BEET GREENS (leaves and stems, cooked, drained)	1 cup	89	trace	trace
BLACK-EYED PEAS (immature seeds, cooked, drained)				
From raw	1 cup	160	1	0.2
From frozen	1 cup	224	1	0.3
BROCCOLI				
Raw				
Chopped or diced	1 cup	25	trace	trace
Spear, 5" long	1 spear	9	trace	trace
Cooked, drained				
From raw				
Chopped	1 cup	44	1	0.1
Spear, 5" long	1 spear	10	trace	trace
From frozen, chopped	1 cup	52	trace	trace
BRUSSELS SPROUTS (cooked, drained)				
From raw	1 cup	61	1	0.2
From frozen	1 cup	65	1	0.1
CABBAGE (common varieties, shredded)				
Raw	1 cup	18	trace	trace
Cooked, drained	1 cup	33	1	0.1
CABBAGE, CHINESE (shredded, cooked, drained)				

FOOD	AMOUNT	CALORIES	FAT (G)	SATURATED FAT (G)
PAK CHOI / BOK CHOY	1 cup	20	trace	trace
CABBAGE, RED (raw, shredded)	1 cup	19	trace	trace
CABBAGE, SAVOY (raw, shredded)	1 cup	19	trace	trace
CARROT JUICE, CANNED	1 cup	94	trace	0.1
CARROTS				
Raw				
Whole, 7½" long	1 carrot	31	trace	trace
Grated	1 cup	47	trace	trace
Baby	1 medium	4	trace	trace
Cooked, sliced, drained				
From raw	1 cup	70	trace	0.1
From frozen	1 cup	53	trace	trace
Canned, sliced, drained	1 cup	37	trace	0.1
CAULIFLOWER				
Raw	1 floret	3	trace	trace
	1 cup	25	trace	trace
CELERY				
Raw				
Stalk, 8" long	1 stalk	6	trace	trace
Pieces, diced	1 cup	19	trace	trace
CHIVES, RAW	1 tbsp.	1	trace	trace
CILANTRO, RAW	1 tsp.	trace	trace	trace
COLLARDS, COOKED (drained, chopped)				
From raw	1 cup	49	1	0.1
From frozen	1 cup	61	1	0.1
CORN, SWEET, YELLOW				
Cooked, drained				
From raw cob	1 ear	83	1	0.2
From frozen				
Kernels on cob	1 ear	59	trace	0.1
Kernels	1 cup	131	1	0.1

FOOD	AMOUNT	CALORIES	FAT (G)	SATURATED FAT (G)
Canned				
Cream style	1 cup	184	1	0.2
Whole kernel, vacuum pack	1 cup	166	1	0.2
CUCUMBER				
Peeled				
Sliced	1 cup	14	trace	trace
Whole, 8¼"	1 large	34	trace	0.1
Unpeeled				
Sliced	1 cup	14	trace	trace
Whole, 8¼"	1 large	39	trace	0.1
DILL, RAW	5 sprigs	trace	trace	trace
EGGPLANT (cooked, drained)	1 cup	28	trace	trace
GARLIC, RAW	1 clove	4	trace	trace
KALE (cooked, drained, chopped)				
From raw	1 cup	36	1	0.1
From frozen	1 cup	39	1	0.1
LEEKS, (bulb and lower leaf, chopped, cooked, drained)	1 cup	32	trace	trace
LETTUCE, RAW				
Butterhead, Boston types				
Leaf	1 medium leaf	1	trace	trace
Head, 5" diameter	1 head	21	trace	trace
Crisphead, as iceberg				
Leaf	1 medium	1	trace	trace
Head, 6" diameter	1 head	65	1	0.1
Pieces, shredded or chopped	1 cup	7	trace	trace
Loose leaf head				
Leaf	1 leaf	2	trace	trace
Pieces, shredded	1 cup	10	trace	trace
Romaine or Cos				
Inner leaf	1 leaf	1	trace	trace
Pieces, shredded	1 cup	8	trace	trace

FOOD	AMOUNT	CALORIES	FAT (G)	SATURATED FAT (G)
MUSHROOMS				
Raw, cut up	1 cup	18	trace	trace
Cooked, drained	1 cup	42	1	0.1
Canned, drained	1 cup	37	trace	0.1
MUSHROOMS, SHIITAKE				
Cooked pieces	1 cup	80	trace	0.1
Dried	1 mushroom	11	trace	trace
MUSTARD GREENS (cooked, drained)	1 cup	21	trace	trace
OKRA (sliced, cooked, drained)				
From raw	1 cup	51	trace	0.1
From frozen	1 cup	52	1	0.1
ONIONS				
Raw				
Chopped	1 cup	61	trace	trace
Whole, medium, 2½" diameter	1 whole	42	trace	trace
Slice, ⅛" thick	1 slice	5	trace	trace
Cooked (whole or sliced), drained	1 cup	92	trace	0.1
	1 medium	41	trace	trace
Dehydrated flakes	1 tbsp.	17	trace	trace
PARSLEY, RAW	10 sprigs	4	trace	trace
PARSNIPS (sliced, cooked, drained)	1 cup	126	trace	0.1
PEAS (edible pod, cooked, drained)				
From raw	1 cup	67	trace	0.1
From frozen	1 cup	83	1	0.1
PEAS, GREEN				
Canned, drained	1 cup	117	1	0.1
Frozen	1 cup	125	trace	0.1
PEPPERS				
Hot chili, raw				
Green	1 pepper	18	trace	trace
Red	1 pepper	18	trace	trace

FOOD	AMOUNT	CALORIES	FAT (G)	SATURATED FAT (G)
Jalapeño, canned, sliced, solids and liquids	¼ cup	7	trace	trace
Sweet (2¾" long, 2½" diameter)				
Raw				
Green				
Chopped	1 cup	40	trace	trace
Whole	1 pepper	32	trace	trace
Red				
Chopped	1 cup	40	trace	trace
Whole	1 pepper	32	trace	trace
Cooked, drained, chopped				
Green	1 cup	38	trace	trace
Red	1 cup	38	trace	trace
POTATOES				
Baked (2⅓" x 4¾")				
With skin	1 potato	220	trace	0.1
Flesh only	1 potato	145	trace	trace
Boiled (2½" diameter)				
Peeled after boiling	1 potato	118	trace	trace
Peeled before boiling	1 potato	116	trace	trace
	1 cup	134	trace	trace
POTATO PRODUCTS (prepared)				
From dry mix, with whole milk, butter	1 cup	228	10	6.3
From home recipe, with butter	1 cup	323	19	11.6
Fried, frozen, oven-heated	10 strips	10	4	0.6
Hashed brown				
From frozen (about 3" x 1½" x ½")	1 patty	63	3	1.3
From home recipe	1 cup	326	22	8.5
Mashed				
From dehydrated flakes (milk, butter, salt added)	1 cup	237	12	7.2
From home recipe				
With whole milk	1 cup	162	1	0.7

FOOD	AMOUNT	CALORIES	FAT (G)	SATURATED FAT (G)
With whole milk and margarine	1 cup	223	9	2.2
Potato salad, (home-prepared)	1 cup	358	21	3.6
Scalloped				
From dry mix, with whole milk, butter	1 cup	228	11	6.5
From home recipe, with butter	1 cup	211	9	5.5
PUMPKIN				
Cooked, mashed	1 cup	49	trace	0.1
Canned	1 cup	83	1	0.4
RADISHES, RAW	1 radish	1	trace	trace
RUTABAGAS, COOKED	1 cup	66	trace	trace
SAUERKRAUT (canned, solids and liquid)	1 cup	45	race	0.1
SEAWEED				
Kelp, raw	2 tbsp.	4	trace	trace
Spirulina, dried	1 tbsp.	3	trace	trace
SHALLOTS, CHOPPED	1 tbsp.	7	trace	trace
SOYBEANS, GREEN (cooked, drained)	1 cup	254	12	1.3
SPINACH				
Raw				
Chopped	1 cup	7	trace	trace
Leaf	1 leaf	2	trace	trace
Cooked, drained				
From raw	1 cup	41	trace	0.1
From frozen (chopped or leaf)	1 cup	53	trace	0.1
Canned, drained	1 cup	49	1	0.2
SQUASH				
Summer (all varieties), sliced, cooked, drained	1 cup	36	1	0.1
Winter (all varieties), baked, cubes	1 cup	80	1	0.3
SWEET POTATOES				
Cooked (2" diameter, 5" long raw)				
Baked, with skin	1 potato	150	trace	trace
Boiled, without skin	1 potato	164	race	0.1

FOOD	AMOUNT	CALORIES	FAT (G)	SATURATED FAT (G)
Candied (2½" x 2" piece)	1 piece	144	3	1.4
Canned				
Syrup pack, drained	1 cup	212	1	0.1
Vacuum pack, mashed	1 cup	232	1	0.1
TOMATOES				
Whole	¼" slice	4	trace	trace
Cherry	1 cherry	4	trace	trace
Medium, 2⅗" diameter	1 tomato	26	trace	0.1
Chopped or sliced	1 cup	38	1	0.1
Canned, solids and liquid	1 cup	46	trace	trace
Sun-dried				
Plain	1 piece	5	trace	trace
Packed in oil, drained	1 piece	6	trace	0.1
TOMATO JUICE (canned, salt added)	1 cup	41	trace	trace
TOMATO PRODUCTS (canned)				
Paste	1 cup	215	1	0.2
Purée	1 cup	10	trace	0.1
Sauce	1 cup	74	trace	0.1
Stewed	1 cup	71	trace	trace
TURNIPS, COOKED	1 cup	33	trace	trace
TURNIP GREENS (cooked, drained)				
From raw	1 cup	29	trace	0.1
From frozen	1 cup	49	1	0.2
VEGETABLES, MIXED				
Canned, drained	1 cup	77	trace	0.1
Frozen, cooked	1 cup	107	trace	0.1

MISCELLANEOUS ITEMS

HUMMUS, PREPARED	1 tbsp.	23	1	0.2
MAYONNAISE				
Regular	1 tbsp.	99	11	1.6

FOOD	AMOUNT	CALORIES	FAT (G)	SATURATED FAT (G)
Fat-free	1 tbsp.	12	trace	0.1
MUSTARD, YELLOW	1 tsp.	3	trace	trace
OLIVES, CANNED				
Pickled, green	5 medium	20	2	0.3
Ripe, black	5 large	25	2	0.3
PICKLES (cucumber)				
Dill, whole, medium	1 pickle	12	trace	trace
Bread-and-butter slices, 1½" diameter, ¼" thick	3 slices	18	trace	trace
Pickle relish, sweet	1 tbsp.	20	trace	trace
PORK SKINS/RINDS (plain)	1 oz.	155	9	3.2
POTATO CHIPS				
Regular				
Plain				
Salted	1 oz.	152	10	3.1
Barbecue flavor	1 oz.	139	9	2.3
Sour cream and onion-flavored	1 oz.	151	10	2.5
Reduced-fat	1 oz.	134	6	1.2
Made from dried potatoes				
Plain	1 oz.	158	11	2.7
Sour cream and onion-flavored	1 oz.	155	10	2.7
Reduced-fat	1 oz.	142	7	1.5
SOY PRODUCTS				
Soy milk	1 cup	81	5	0.5
Tofu				
Firm	¼ block	62	4	0.5
Soft, piece 2½" x ½" x 1"	1 piece	73	4	0.6
TRAIL MIX				
Regular (raisins, chocolate chips, salted nuts, seeds)	1 cup	707	47	8.9
Tropical	1 cup	570	24	11.9

Essential Vitamins & Minerals
Five Great Sources for Your Daily Essentials[4]

DIETARY FIBER

The recommended daily allowance for adult women is 25 grams.

FOOD	AMOUNT	DIETARY FIBER (G)
Navy beans, cooked	½ cup	9.5
Split peas, cooked	½ cup	8.1
Lentils, cooked	½ cup	7.8
Lima beans, cooked	½ cup	6.6
Artichoke, cooked	1 globe	6.5

CALCIUM

The recommended daily allowance for adults is 1,000 milligrams.

FOOD	AMOUNT	DIETARY FIBER (G)
Plain yogurt, non-fat	8 oz.	452
Romano cheese	1.5 oz.	452
Swiss cheese	1.5 oz.	335
Provolone cheese	1.5 oz.	321
Cheddar cheese	1.5 oz.	307

4. Information taken from "Dietary Guidelines for Americans 2010"
   U.S. Department of Health and Human Services
   U.S. Department of Agriculture
   www.health.gov/dietaryguidelines/dga2010/DietaryGuidelines2010.pdf

IRON

The recommended daily allowance for teen and adult females is 18 milligrams.

FOOD	AMOUNT	DIETARY FIBER (G)
Clams, canned, drained	3 oz.	23.8
Oysters, eastern wild, cooked	3 oz.	10.2
Soybeans, mature, cooked	½ cup	4.4
Pumpkin and squash seed kernels, roasted	1 oz.	4.2
White beans, canned	½ cup	3.9

POTASSIUM

The recommended daily allowance for adults is 4,700 milligrams.

FOOD	AMOUNT	DIETARY FIBER (G)
Sweet potato, baked	1 potato (146 g)	694
Beet greens, cooked	½ cup	655
Potato, baked, flesh	1 potato (156 g)	610
White beans, canned	½ cup	595
Yogurt, plain, non-fat	8 oz.	579

VITAMIN A

The recommended daily allowance of Vitamin A for adult men is 900 micrograms.

FOOD	AMOUNT	VITAMIN A (MICROGRAMS)
Carrot juice	¾ cup	1,692
Sweet potato w/peel, baked	1 medium	1,096
Pumpkin, canned	½ cup	953
Carrots, cooked from fresh	½ cup	671
Spinach, cooked from frozen	½ cup	573

VITAMIN C

The recommended daily allowance of Vitamin C for adult men is 90 milligrams.

FOOD	AMOUNT	VITAMIN C (MG)
Guava, raw	½ cup	188
Red sweet pepper, raw	½ cup	142
Klwl fruit	1 medium	70
Orange juice	¾ cup	61–93
Grapefruit juice	¾ cup	50–70

ESSENTIAL VITAMINS AND MINERALS

VITAMIN E

The recommended daily allowance of Vitamin E for adults is 15 milligrams.

FOOD	AMOUNT	VITAMIN E (MG)
Sunflower seeds, dry roasted	1 oz.	7.4
Almonds	1 oz.	7.3
Sunflower oil	1 tbsp.	5.6
Hazelnuts (filberts)	1 oz.	4.3
Mixed nuts, dry-roasted	1 oz.	3.1